SELF MASTERY FOR HEALTH

How to Transform Your Health And Life In 6 Simple Steps

by DR. STEPHANIE KABONGO

Moringa Better Life Ltd
No 6 Doreen Street,
Colbyn, Pretoria
0083, South Africa

Disclaimer

The information provided in this book is designed to provide helpful information on the subjects discussed. This book is not meant to be used, nor should it be used, to diagnose or treat any medical condition. For diagnosis or treatment of any medical problem, consult your own physician.

The publisher and author are not responsible for any specific medical or health needs that may require supervision by a licensed healthcare practitioner, and thus they are not liable for any consequences from any recommendation, to any person reading or following the information in this book.

Photographer: Linda Bell +855 12 774 214 (office@belatel.com), location Auckland New Zealand.

Contents

Dr. Stephanie Kabongo

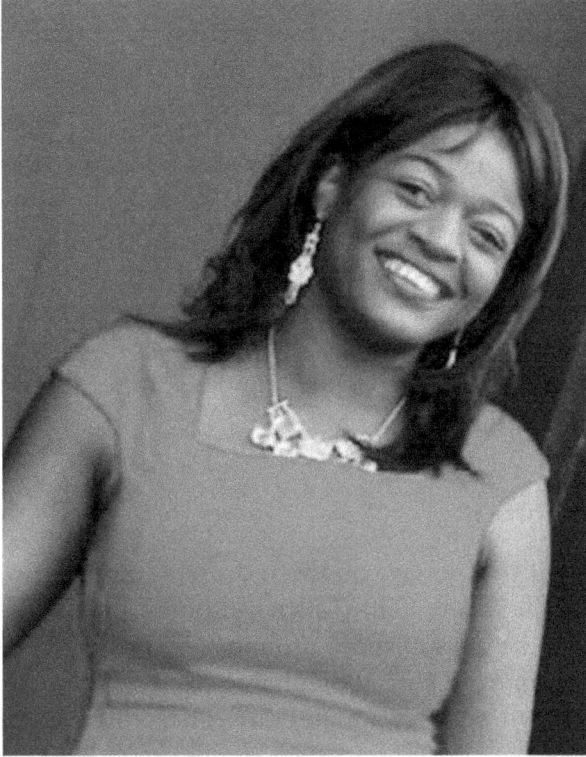

Meet Dr. Stephanie K

Dr. Stephanie K is a medical doctor who also works as a health and a success coach. Her passion for helping people succeed in losing weight, getting healthy, and achieving their goals in life is well recognized because Stephanie understands the struggles of her clients, as she had to overcome many huge obstacles in her own life.

After struggling to get through medical school in a tough, racially-charged university, then immigrating as an African woman to a new country far away from the support of her friends and family where life was less than ideal, it took a great deal of mind-setting to get to where she is today, but Stephanie did it. No stranger to hard work and overcoming challenges, today, Dr. Stephanie K uses her own personal experience to motivate her coaching clients and her seminar audiences to achieve more in their lives.

Her Realization…

The pivotal point that set her on the right path occurred when she was forced to see life in a new light. Taken out of her perspective and forced to look through the eyes of those around her who were worse off than she was, this awareness is what Stephanie credits for the success she has today, both her own, and the one she helps others discover for themselves.

It all started while Stephanie was laid up in a hospital bed, after a routine operation from an old hip injury. Looking back on it now, Dr. Stephanie Kabongo thinks of that life-changing insight as an 'Oprah moment' of sorts.

Recalling her time as a patient, Stephanie describes her experience in that hospital as one of the lowest points in her life. Until then, she was used to being the doctor. Now she was the patient lying on the bed and waiting for the doctors to do their ward rounds. It was a strange role reversal which turned out to be a real enlightening experience she never expected.

It was a new hospital, and they had forgotten to put her title "Dr." before her name. That little mistake gave her the advantage, allowing her to see what was like to be treated just like every other patient in the hospital. It was a shock.

During these ward rounds, Stephanie felt as if the ticking clock was more important than she was as a patient. In hospitals, ward rounds are usually done pretty quickly, to make sure each patient is seen to.

As is the standard procedure, when the Doctors arrived at Stephanie's bedside, they pulled back the curtain, talked to each other about her post-operation status, and then removed the bandage from her large surgical wound. After looking at it and commenting to each other that it was healing well, they left. What they didn't do was talk to her, only among themselves and before leaving.

To her, the whole experience was very strange now that the tables were turned, and she could see how impersonal it actually was.

It was shocking to see them just walk away, without taking the time to talk to her as a patient or as a human being, a person coping with the wound they were examining. Again, without conferring with the patient, the doctors ordered the nurse to instruct physiotherapy to come take 'the wounded patient' to rehab and then get her discharged home in two days. That was that.

They talked *about* her as if she wasn't even there in the bed in front of them, being examined.

All in all, Stephanie was shocked at their insensitivity. This was a real eye opener. Her mouth went dry, and she couldn't speak because she was so aghast at how badly this must come across to all patients in general. She often talks about this saying:

> *"As a hospital doctor myself, I had been doing ward rounds just like those doctors who saw me. In my moment in that hospital bed, I was shocked and disgusted at how it felt to be their patient. In that life- changing moment, I made my decision never to treat patients in that way. I committed to always have a holistic approach to patient care, which considers their feelings and wellness."*

This role reversal incident indeed reawakened the doctor/healer inside Stephanie as to what it feels like to be a patient under her own care. She describes this as feeling totally worthless as a human being.

In that moment, Dr. Stephanie realized she never wanted to make anybody feel as terrible as she did that day, and that she could give more, go deeper and help people heal in ways that honoured them as whole, loving and complete beings. She made a decision then to begin a journey that would change her life and the lives of her patients and clients.

Dr. Stephanie Kabongo is a leading authority on health and success breakthroughs. She will teach you how to achieve your success and a stress-free life... no matter your starting point.

No people won't be required to read her books before doing the trainings but it will be recommended.

Preface

After that traumatic time at the hospital and feeling little better than a number on a form, Stephanie decided to change her focus to help others achieve their ultimate in personal success, health and well-being through holistic success coaching and natural health care.

Her journey as a well-respected MD included a special interest in health and wellness related to stress management. Her study of the effects of stress on the human body and the mind has led her to further education in Public Health, nutritional medicine, natural hormones, anti-aging and regenerative medicine.

Stephanie uses natural alternatives wherever possible, including health coaching, Bio-Identical Hormones, organic herbs and supplements. She is passionate about people's success, health and happiness.

"I discovered that empowering people to succeed in life, improves their health and energy levels. It gives me the greatest satisfaction in my career and in my life to witness that occurring."

Dr. Stephanie's core mission is to help people eliminate struggle, failures and un-healthiness from their lives and to be successful and stress-free! She works with clients on achieving success, losing weight, stress-related conditions, hormone imbalance, anxiety disorders, burn-out, adrenal fatigue, etc. With her help, her clients are able to overcome their struggles, their stress, and burn-out with simple and effective techniques. They regain their health, success, happiness, and vitality.

One of the ways she does this is through one on one coaching, group coaching, mastermind groups, and live events where she inspires others to transform their lives.

As a trained medical doctor, she has a vast knowledge of the effects of stress on the human body such as hormonal balance, mental disorders, and more. She uses her medical resources to the client's advantage and satisfaction, and helps them lose weight the natural and holistic way.

Dedication

This book is dedicated first to the deep gratitude I have for Almighty God, the Creator of all and to His son, my Lord and Saviour Jesus Christ.

I am grateful for my ability to motivate, inspire and communicate these health and success coaching lessons that I've discovered through my natural medicine career and through consistent study of self-development teachings, books and seminars.

I also dedicate this book to my loving, caring and supportive family and friends, as well as to those who are struggling to succeed in health or life goals.

My final dedication is to those who choose to persist, and refuse to accept failure or to settle for less than they deserve. This is for all the men and women who know that they deserve success and who are willing to keep learning new ways to succeed in their lives, despite all odds. Success is coming, and it will meet you on your way! You are closer than you think! Keep the faith alive! Never give up!

Introduction

To my beautiful friends, I first want to thank you and congratulate you for buying my book. Not every day you discover a book that teaches you how to appreciate yourself, your health and your success, no matter your stage in life.

By reading this book and applying what you learn, you'll change the way you view your body, the way you view your health, and will simplify your path to success. Let me begin with the concept of:

Every aspect of you is interconnected...

You are the common denominator in your health, your success, your relationships, and in everything in your entire life. By reading this book, you will view yourself in a completely new way; one that you probably have not seen before. After reading this book, you will feel a different connection to your body, an improved connection to your success and an enlightened connection to your environment.

The only thing I ask is that you have a relaxed approach as you read the book, extract what resonates with you, and apply it to your new way of doing and being.

This book doesn't discriminate against anyone or anything. It is written to unite all who are looking forward to succeeding with health and life goals. It's written so that anyone can enjoy making the changes in their daily life that are supportive of improved health, well-being and success.

Improvements can begin in anyone's life, no matter if they are the leader of the pack, or the last in a line of wannabes. One key to remember is it's not how you start that matters... but THAT you start – that is what's important.

We all have the ability to succeed in everything we set our minds to accomplish in our lives... without exception. Health is simply a success goal just like any other, and all success goals are absolutely achievable.

Attaining great health is your innate birth right. It is not a "reserved only table" for the special ones. It is within reach of all of us. Even though many people fail at the success goals of money, good health and weight loss, I believe that with more knowledge and the empowerment of principles, that can easily change.

Self Mastery for Health

Self Mastery Health empowers you with a winning mind-set to tackle any success goal, including health and losing weight. It's not just limited to health; the principles can be applied to career choices and all relationships in your life.

The Importance of Getting the Proper Mind-set and Clarity

Without the right mind-set, you'll struggle forever with attempts at achieving anything and everything. One of the first things you have to get right -- is a winning mind-set, *your* winning mind-set.

> *If weight loss is your goal, then I suggest you apply the principles that are believable and suitable for you.*

Some techniques that you'll learn with me will put you in a space of knowing what you really want to achieve in life. You'll become clearer and more focused on your success goals. Once you have that clarity, and I truly believe that clarity is power (more on that later), many of you will achieve more of your goals because you are becoming absolutely clear as to exactly what those goals are.

Even your attitude and associations relating to your goals must change in order to change the outcomes of your goals. You are truly the only one who can easily make your success goals reality. Other people may guide you, but at the end of the day, the life journey on that path of success is yours alone to take. This book is simply a guide book along that path; one that will provide more empowerment for your ability to succeed.

What inspired me to write this book?

Inspiration for this book came to me as I discovered myself repeating the same concepts to my clients as I helped them lose weight, succeed in their career goals, or heal from chronic diseases naturally.

It is a rule of mine that no matter what success or health goal we want to achieve, there are always solutions hidden in our lives and environments that can help us get there.

I always give my clients very simple explanations regarding their body's physiology, and tell them that there is a hidden wisdom resident within everyone's bodies. Then, it dawned on me that I could put all that wisdom into a book to help everyone achieve best results in their lives.

If my clients could make better life choices based on the information they were taking away from our sessions, then it made sense that others could also benefit from reading about these concepts.

Self Mastery Health is a way to reunite us all with the understanding we are all in the same boat when it comes to our health. We have all struggled with one health issue or another.

The need to lose weight is as common a denominator as the common cold. All of us who tried so many different ways to get healthy know what a daunting task it can be to keep trying to lose while stuck at the same weight. Or, it could be even worse... gaining weight instead of losing. The same concern applies to other forms of success that we try so hard to achieve in life, only to end up with greater failures.

This book is for all who never really learned how to succeed. Everyone has an idea of what it is, but we do not have a clue how to attain it and keep it in our daily, busy, stressed and hectic lives. We often disassociate ourselves from success as if it is "out there" or a "too hard, not for me" thing. Some of us have not learned that being successful, healthy and living at our ideal weight is not a privilege for only a few, but **it is our birth right to have**! In simple terms – **You Were Born To Win!** This book is for all who are expected to know far more than they know, and really need to recognize how to access success. If there is a vulnerable person freaking out about their lack of success, this book will rapidly and dramatically change their circumstance.

In the past, these folks did not know what to do and often have settled for less. That's ok, that's in the past – and remember it's never too late to turn your life around for the better.

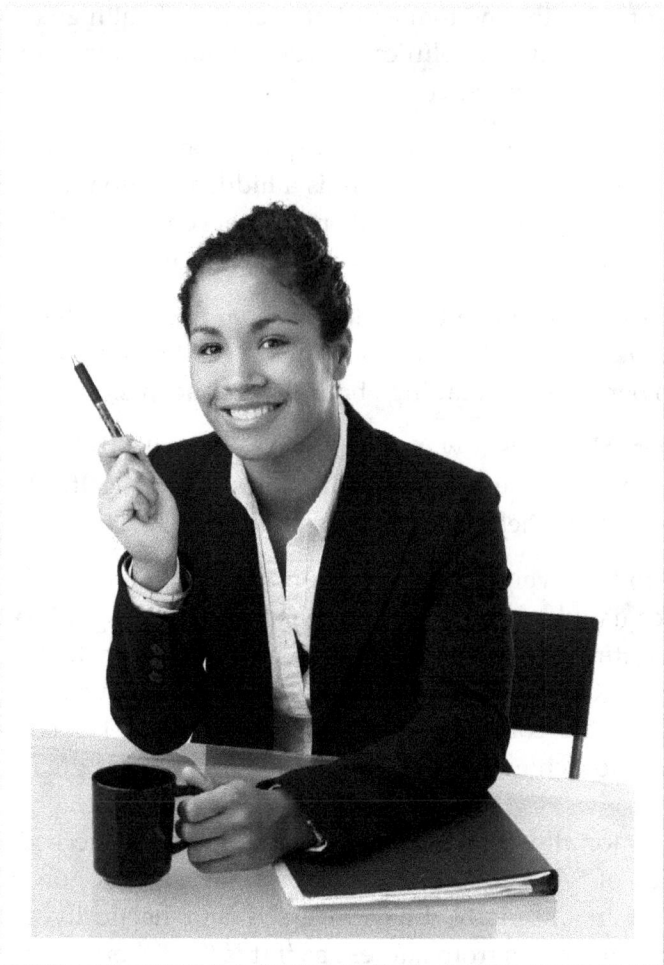

CHAPTER I

A Successful Healthy Body

Your embodiment of success

Your body consists of more than 47 trillion cells. These cells developed from the fertilization of ONE sperm and ONE egg (from your mother and your father). Once those two cells joined, they formed a single cell that was the beginning of you.

That single cell then divided into two, and those two cells in turn divided into four, and divided from four into eight. They continued dividing themselves exponentially. Then, at some point, your cells started specializing in different tissues and organs such as muscle, stomach, heart and bones. After nine months, the miracle happens… a new being enters the world.

The body you live in today is different from the body that you had when you were a baby because, of course, you grew. The human body is always in the process of growing and replacing its cells. All the cells in your body are programmed to have a limited lifespan, after which they are discarded and replaced by brand new cells. This is why you look different from the way you looked at the age of 2, 10 or 18 years.

Even as an adult, your cells still are going through their growth cycle and are being replaced by new cells as they exhaust their lives.

The cells in your body are renewed and are replaced at different rates, for example:

- Your white blood cells are replaced every day,
- Your stomach cells are replaced every two days,
- Your colon cells every four days,
- Your skin cells every 3-6 weeks, and
- Your bone cells every 25 years.

Only your brain and nervous system are never replaced; they are simply repaired as best as they can. Therefore, every year, apart from the bones and nerve cells, you have a brand new physical body.

That is good news for health, healing, or even for weight loss. It means that whatever is going on in your body right now has the potential to change naturally. You have the ability to create better living cells in your body simply by allowing the natural renewal process to take place in a healthier environment and with enhanced support for your body. If you change a few things about how you are looking after your body, such as a better nutrition, your new cells will be of better quality and health. Isn't this good news? This is very important to understand as it plays a big role in your ability to avoid diseases or to lose weight.

However, here comes the catch. In order for the cells in your body to replicate themselves, they need good-quality building materials. This is where good nutrition comes in. The food you eat provides nutrition, which the body uses to rebuild itself. You do not just eat for the sake of eating. You eat to provide your body with raw materials to rebuild you all over again. You become exactly what you have eaten before. The protein you eat is used for structures such as muscles, the fat you eat becomes part of the cell walls, and carbohydrates become energy.

As cells divide constantly, they group together into tissues, which then join to form organs such as your heart, lungs and stomach. Your heart is an organ made up of specialized tissue cells that function differently from the tissue cells of your lungs or your brain.

Oneness in your body

Even though the different parts of your body have specialized functions, they still collaborate and work together in unison. When this happens across all parts of your body, both internally and externally, there is perfect health. Externally you have a head, two arms and two legs. These body parts have unique and specialized functions that they perform every day of your life. Your legs take you from point A to point B; your arms carry things; your eyes see things, and your nose breathes and smells things. Every part works independently while also collaborating with the rest.

Every part is so super specialized in its task that it will never cross over to do another function different from the one it does well. For example, your eyes cannot change from seeing to smelling; only your nose can smell. Your legs will only move you around and get you to your destination. They will not suddenly start carrying things for you, only your arms can do that well. Your arms are more than happy to do what they are specialized to do. Just by looking at your external body parts, you can see that your body has various essential elements that are designed for a specific function.

There is no shortcut when it comes to your knowledge of the body parts and their roles and duties. Therefore, what you call your body is the sum of all those parts working together in harmony. You can have a look at your hands, your feet, your ears, your eyes, and realize that you are made up of many parts that are important, efficient and specialized. Just the external parts of your body are worth being appreciated for what they do for you. Learn to be grateful daily for what your body does with total and complete ease. Being healthy is not just about losing weight and fitting into skinny jeans. It is about having your body functioning well enough to keep you living your life.

The same goes for your internal systems. Your stomach has a specialized and precise role that it plays all day long. Your heart beats continuously and sends blood through your body. Your lungs breathe all day and all night. Your internal organs are super specialized; they know their roles to precision. Your heart will never suddenly become so confused about its job that it will harm you deliberately. Your organs are so unique in their functioning and daily tasks that they resemble a symphony orchestra, where every instrument is singular, highly developed and precise. Every organ in your body influences the other. There is no division or isolation. When your lungs breathe in oxygen from the air, that oxygen meets the blood coming from your heart. The oxygen being taken up by your blood is exchanged for carbon dioxide, which is returned to your lungs and exhaled into the atmosphere. This whole process happens as you breathe in and breathe out. Your heart sends blood to your lungs to release its carbon dioxide content into the lungs, and then in return it brings the oxygen exchanged from the lungs back to the heart. Your heart then beats again and sends the new blood containing oxygen through your blood vessels to your entire body, to your tissues and cells. As you can see, the two organs are specific in their functions but work together in fantastic collaboration. Next time you take a breath, remember that your heart and lungs are collaborating to purify and circulate your blood.

My point is that you need to start realizing the connections that exist in your body and be grateful for what it does for you. Your body parts are not just there accidentally; they are as precise as precise can be. Every part of you is you. There are your fingers, your ankles, your fat belly, and your thunder thighs. Every bit of you is just that... it is YOU. Your internal organ system is the same; everything works independently but joins in harmony to keep you healthy. When you put too much stress on one of your body parts or organs, you end up with disease.

When the symptoms of disease and un-wellness start to be manifest, your body tries to compensate. It uses other parts and organs but cannot manage, so now it requires support. Your symptoms or un-wellness is not just a way for your body to bother you. Your body is creating awareness that the way you are living is overwhelming and is stressing an organ or a part of it. Your symptoms are a wake-up call to change something that you are doing to your body. Even gaining weight is simply a warning sign from your body that your current lifestyle is not good for you.

Your body is magnificent. Everything from the internal to the external aspects of it is purposefully placed and mastered. Everything functions together. No function is more important than the other is. The body sees your little toe as important as your head or heart. You will go into protection mode if something is dropped on your little toe just as much as if something is dropped on your head. Your body has the concept that everything is one thing, and one thing is everything, as far as its parts and organs are concerned. If you are talking to your friend and an insect crawls up your foot, you will take your attention away from your friend and deal with the insect. You will remove it from your foot no matter how important your conversation is. Every part of you is independent and yet dependent on the running of the whole body. There is no division in the body, each part of it is and has an equal power. It is important to remember that if one organ or part of your body is suffering, it will eventually start to affect the other parts. The opposite applies, if one part is honored every part rejoices.

When embarking on a new journey of adventure with your body, remember it never works any of its parts in isolation. Everything is always together. Remember, one thing is everything and everything is one thing. Becoming healthier or going on a weight loss journey cannot be done in isolation. Slimming down your body or becoming healthier is not an isolative thing.

Trying to lose weight and become healthier has a lot to do with your cardiovascular and digestive system. As discussed before, no single system works in isolation. The improvement of one system's functions will affect the others towards a more holistic health revival in your body.

As you start to appreciate your body, you begin to notice how your body sustains you daily living, how it does so much for you. You start feeling gratitude for your body. It breathes for you and carries you to where you want to go. Your body allows you to read this book; it allows you to watch that movie, and allows you to enjoy eating delicious food. What would you be like without your body? The change of self-image will lead you very quickly to be grateful daily for the work your body does for you, that you are not even aware of. It is such a humbling experience to think that at any second, there is so much going on in your body that is keeping you alive! My clients often are humbled when I tell them that a new self-image is crucial to the well-functioning of their body and therefore, their wellness as a whole.

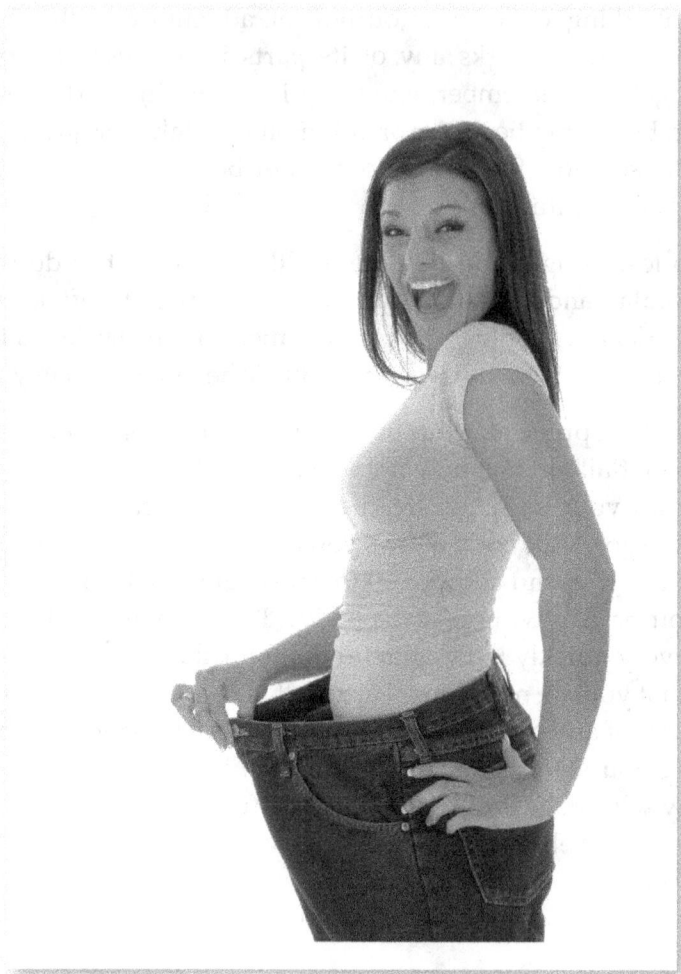

CHAPTER 2

Successful Weight Loss

This book is about helping you understand how being healthy really works. Digestion is an important system because it is how your body acquires the nutrition it needs. The Self Mastery for Health combine to gift you total health, but digestion dominates the physical component. The foods you eat will do nothing for you if they are not digested properly and adequately. The Chinese and Ayurvedic medicine practitioners believe that all diseases have their root cause in poor digestion. I agree with them. Many people have poor digestive systems that cause them discomfort, either directly or indirectly.

The third step in getting your Self Mastery for Health is to improve your digestion, which ultimately holds the key to unlocking your health and wellness. All the good food in the world will not help if your body is not working properly and absorbing the nutrients you are giving it. The opposite also applies. When your digestive system is functioning optimally, you are absorbing every nutrient from your food and swimming in the sea of health. A good flowing system is a gift you need to give your body regularly, and the rewards are amazing. When you treat this part of your body well, it treats you well in return and enables the proper functioning of your other organs. Since your digestive system influences 70% of your immune system, poor absorption and breakdown lead directly to a weak immune system. This increases the chance of diseases in your body. Therefore, it is imperative to look after your digestion for disease prevention.

The digestive system is connected to all the other systems in your body. It even affects your mood. Have you ever noticed how eating a good meal lifts up your mood, or how people seek comfort in food? Some healers are convinced that this system is our "second brain," and the second most important in our body. Just like our brain, our gut also releases the chemical serotonin, a neurotransmitter that makes you happy, calm and content.

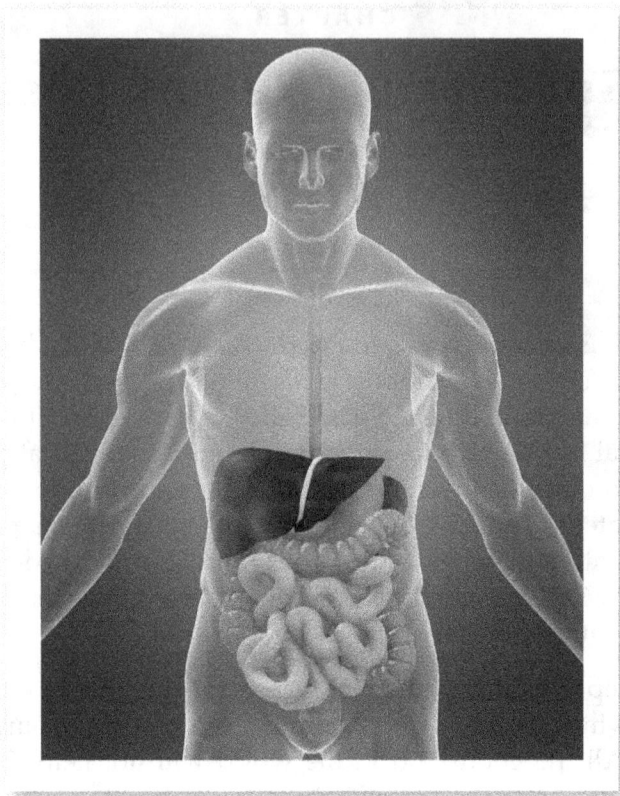

CHAPTER 3

How Digestion Works

Many people have digestive problems. Some have difficulties digesting certain foods. Regardless of your health level or in what diet theory you believe, we can all agree that we need to improve our digestion to keep being healthy.

Whether you want to lose weight or just simply be healthier, you need to have a basic knowledge of how your body digests food for health and energy. I am going to give you a simple lesson on how the body digests and absorbs the food we eat every day.

Digestion is the breaking down of food into small enough components that the body absorbs. Once the food has been broken down, nutrients are extracted and distributed into the body for nourishment.

When you take a piece of food, chew it and swallow, it goes through all the organs of your digestive system. When it moves through the lining of your digestive tract and into your bloodstream, that is when you actually absorb the nutrients.

Absorption is the movement of nutrients, including water and electrolytes, across the intestinal wall and into your bloodstream.

The digestive system includes your mouth, pharynx, esophagus, stomach, pancreas, liver, gall bladder and both your small and large intestines. It does not act alone; it is part of all the other bodily systems, and they all collaborate with each other. It needs all the systems of the body to work properly.

Your endocrine system secretes all your hormones. Your nervous system sends signals from your brain down through your body, and controls your hunger and the passage and absorption of food, while your cardiovascular system transports all the nutrients through your bloodstream once they are absorbed. Then the urinary or elimination system gets rid of the waste products of digestion.

All your systems are super-specialized in their functions, and all work together in perfect harmony. When there is collaboration, there is health. You need every part of your body to be working well to utilize the nutrients from the food that you eat.

The digestive tract is a hollow tube about 30 feet in length, which runs from the mouth to the anus. The transit time for food through the whole system can be anywhere from 24 to 72 hours. Many things affect the time that food takes to go through your system. It can be the composition of your meal, physical activity, emotions, the medications you may be taking, or any illnesses.

The way you digest your food may vary from time to time as well. There are also important secretions from glands that are necessary to make the whole process work.

For example, there is mucous, which is important for moistening, lubricating and protecting the lining of your entire digestive tract. There are digestive enzymes that work in every aspect of your body. The enzymes are catalysts that cause reactions. Enzymes are protein molecules that the digestive system uses to break down food. They are secreted by the mouth, the pancreas, and the small intestine to aid the whole process.

You also have hormones involved in this process, as mentioned above. The hormones are chemical messengers secreted into the blood by a gland that regulates the body's functioning.

Underneath the mucosal lining of our stomach is the lymphatic tissue, and this tissue is our immune system. The most common way that foreign bodies enter our system is through the mouth, with what we eat. Our immune system needs to be there with the lymphatic tissue of the stomach to check everything out and make sure things are ok, assessing good and bad all the time.

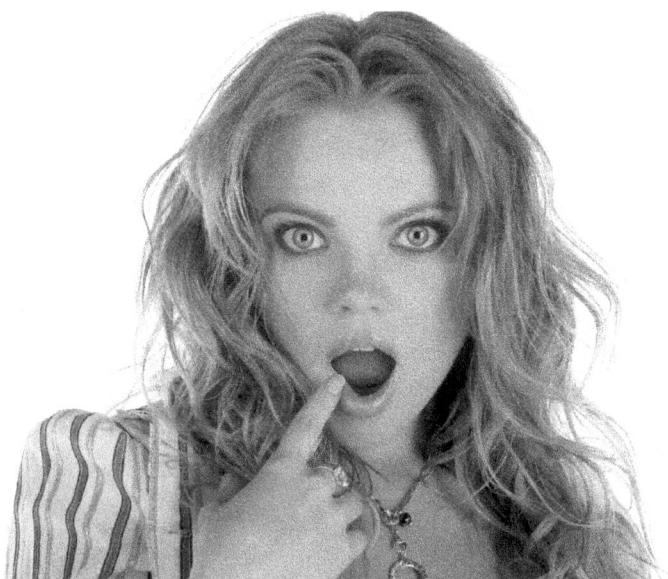

CHAPTER 4

Mouth

The brain is the ultimate commander of the body, so it starts all the processes. Digestion begins even before food enters the mouth. When you smell food or anticipate eating, your brain starts the digestive process. It sends hormone messengers down into the stomach that tells your body to start getting ready for food.

When you smell something cooking and you get that grumbly feeling in your stomach, which is the digestion process beginning. It is anticipating that you are going to eat very soon.

Once food enters your mouth, automatically your teeth start chewing to break the food down into smaller pieces. This is the only part of your digestive tract strong enough to break down the big chunks of food into tinier sizes.

Unfortunately, many people have forgotten how to chew their food properly. They tend to brush the food across their teeth and swallow too quickly. The aim of chewing your food is to have it dissolve into a mash that feels smooth to swallow easily. The way to re-train yourself to chew enough times is to put down your fork between mouthfuls.

Then chew each mouthful 10-20 times before you even consider swallowing it. You have to be conscious while you are eating so that you can focus on what you are doing and how well you are chewing. This takes a bit of practice, but you will get the hang of it.

As you chew, the food mixes with your saliva. Saliva is about 99% water, and the rest is made of a digestive enzyme called amylase, produced by the salivary glands. There is also a pancreatic amylase, which plays a role in digestion further down the process. The salivary amylase enzyme starts the breakdown of carbohydrates in your mouth as you are chewing.

The beauty of digestion is that each type of food has an enzyme that works with it. Therefore, in the case of carbohydrates, amylase is the enzyme that breaks that down. We obviously do not absorb food in the form that we put it into our mouth, so we have to break it down.

When you have a piece of bread, it is made up of complex carbohydrates that consist of long chains of glucose molecules strung together. Your body can only absorb simple carbohydrates in the form of glucose. You have to be able to break down those complex molecules to their simplest form in order to absorb them through the lining of the small intestine. The enzymes get to work and start breaking down complex food into simpler, absorbable forms.

As your tongue rolls the food into a mass, it pushes the food to the back of your throat. When you swallow, the food enters your esophagus, which is a tube about 10 inches long, and is like a pipe that leads to the stomach.

The back of the throat is technically the pharynx, a funnel-shaped opening. It connects the nasal passages and the mouth to your respiratory passages and esophagus. This organ is utilized by both the respiratory tract and the digestive tract.

If you say, "Something went down the wrong pipe" and cough, that is the pharynx not working the way it should. It is allowing the food to go down the respiratory tract instead of the esophagus. No digestion occurs in the esophagus; it is purely for transport. The esophagus has circular muscles all around it, which contract in waves to push down the food.

This process is called "peristalsis" and is a wave-like motion to make things go in the right direction.

TiPS

1. Chew your food well and make sure it mixes properly with the saliva in your mouth.

2. Sit down to eat.

3. Be present and fully conscious when eating.

4. Savor the taste of the food.

5. Say a gratitude prayer.

6. Eat fresh food as much as possible.

7. Minimize the amounts of chewing gum on an empty stomach.

8. Put down your fork between bites to allow for proper chewing. This will help you lose weight, as you will naturally eat less when you chew better.

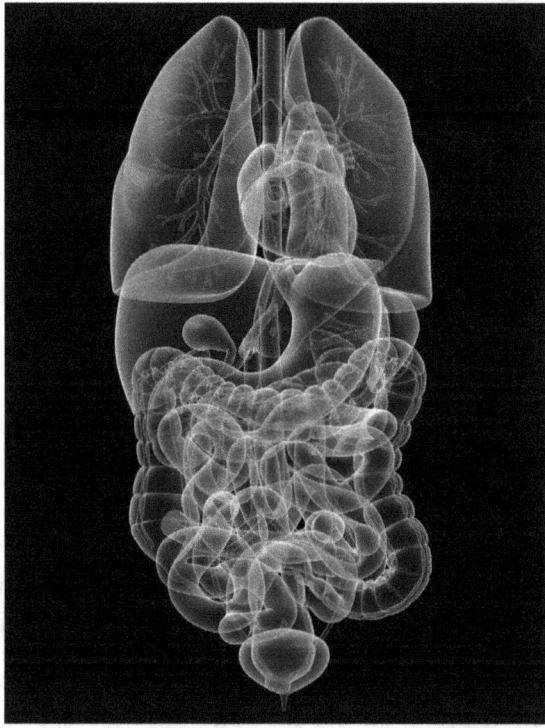

CHAPTER 5

Stomach

The stomach is a 'J' shaped flexible, muscular bag. The top end connects to your esophagus, and the bottom connects to your small intestine.

The upper portion is called a fundus and acts as a reservoir holding food, next feeding it to the lower portion, called the antrum. The stomach is a mixer, so the stomach walls have three layers of muscle that run lengthwise, horizontally and diagonally. They work and contract in different directions: pumping, mixing and pulverizing the food. They mix the food into a soup-like consistency known as chyme.

Therefore, you have the food going down the esophagus and once inside the stomach it mixes with all the enzymes and juices, becoming chyme. The bottom of the stomach is a funnel that slowly empties the chyme into the small intestine. It controls the movement and distribution of the chyme, allowing it to go through gradually.

The only things absorbed in the stomach are alcohol, water and some drugs such as Tylenol. This is why drinking on an empty stomach makes you tipsy quickly.

Also buried in the lining of the stomach are millions of glands that release components of gastric juice. The gastric juice is made up of hydrochloric acid (HCL), and an enzyme called pepsin. Pepsin is one of the enzymes that start the breakdown of protein. The average adult's stomach holds about 2-3 pints of gastric juice, and it is acidic and corrosive enough to strip paint.

The stomach must continually secrete mucous to protect its lining because hydrochloric acid is extremely harsh. The normal pH of the stomach is about 3.5-4.0. When HCL is secreted, it drops that pH to approx. 1-2. Your stomach is the only acidic organ in the body, and it needs to be kept that way to function properly.

Your stomach starts churning automatically when your brain sends a signal, even before you begin eating. When you smell or see food, you get hungry, so the brain tells the stomach to get ready. Hydrochloric acid starts spewing into the stomach, and its muscles start pumping. Even though there is no food, it is ready to go.

That is the growling, gurgling or rumbling you hear. This can become a problem for people who chew gum on an empty stomach. The acids can start to erode the mucous membranes in an empty churning stomach.

Once the food is digested in your stomach, it is ready to be discharged into your intestine for absorption. When you have a full stomach, and the food starts to move into the small intestine, there is a hormone secreted that is called CCK. This hormone signals your pancreas to start releasing its juices. It also signals the release the hormone leptin.

This is the hormone responsible for telling your brain that you are full. This hormone is your best friend because it helps you not to overeat. Unfortunately, many people override this hormone and continue to eat even when they do not have to.

The stomach empties in about 2-6 hours. The length of time can be determined by the size and composition of a meal and even by your emotions. I am interested in how emotions fit into food and eating; it is a fascinating area to me. One of the reasons why I wrote this book was to show people that there is so much more to the body functions than they might think. Everything is always interconnected and inter-related when it comes to you as a being. Our emotions really play a part in how we digest our food.

When it comes to the food composition of a meal, obviously a large meal moves slower than a smaller one. Solid food will move slower than liquid food, while protein moves faster than fat.

Carbohydrates move the quickest, but can be slowed down by the presence of fiber. A mixed meal composed by a protein, a fat, and a carbohydrate takes on average about four hours to empty out of the stomach.

It is interesting how emotions such as sadness and fear can slow down the movement of food, whereas aggression and anger can speed it up. Talking to people about their emotions when they are eating can affect their digestion. Emotional stress causes peptic ulcers that are holes in the stomach lining. One has to be very careful of emotions when digestion is taking place.

TiPS

1. Eat in a quiet area and eat consciously.

2. Keep a tranquil attitude.

3. Avoid heated emotional discussions when eating.

4. Chew well by putting down your fork between bites.

5. Be in a calm state before starting to eat.

6. If you have had poor digestion for a long time, then a spoon of apple cider vinegar before a meal helps your stomach increase its acidity for better digestion.

7. Improve your digestion and improve your health.

8. Weight loss will occur once your body absorbs nutrients properly, so help your stomach help you.

9. A glass of red wine with your meals is allowed (yes, to all my wonderful clients who ask this question).

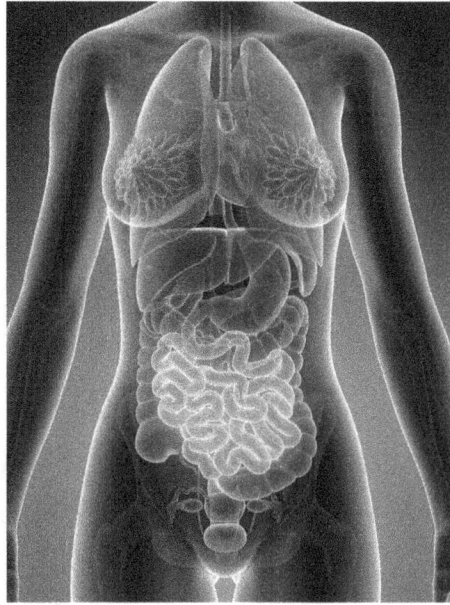

CHAPTER 6

Small Intestine

The small intestine is a long tube about 1 ½ inches in diameter, coiled around beneath your stomach. End to end, an average adult's small intestine is about 22 feet long and is made up of three sections. The duodenum is 12 inches; the jejunum is about 8 feet, and the ileum is about 11 feet.

If the small intestine were simply a tube, it would have an inside surface area of about 4 square yards. In fact, the small intestine is covered with hair-like projections called villi and microvilli that increase the surface area to about 250 square yards.

This is greater than the area of a tennis court. That means you have all that surface area capacity to absorb your food. Your circulatory system lies just underneath the lining of the small intestine. It is through those villi and microvilli that you absorb all the needed nutrients.

The nutrients go straight into your blood system and then blood carries them to the rest of the body. Your body then decides how to use these nutrients.

Your small intestines do their work with the aid of accessory organs. You also have the pancreas, the gall bladder and the liver in the area, and they contribute to further digestion.

Different food components are absorbed in different areas of the small intestine. Carbohydrates, proteins, fat, all the different vitamins, all different minerals, electrolytes and water are absorbed in different areas of the small intestine.

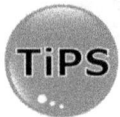

TiPS Minimize your alcohol intake as it interferes with the functioning of your liver. The more congested your liver becomes, the less it contributes to digestion.

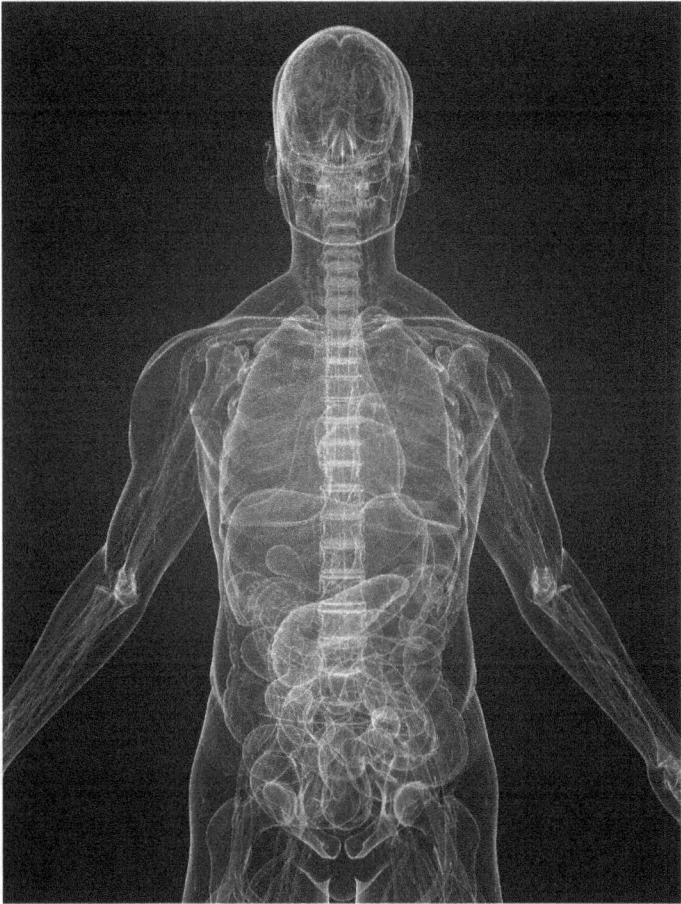

CHAPTER 7

Pancreas

The pancreas is a very small accessory organ with a powerful job. As the chyme leaves your stomach mixed with the acidic gastric juices, the pancreas immediately secretes and sprays bi-carb on it. This brings up the pH to a more neutral level and neutralizes it.

The pancreas is the primary site for digestive enzyme secretion. The enzymes called proteases and lipases are used in the digestion of fats. Those proteases or protein enzymes chop down chains by breaking them into single amino acid and double amino acid units.

That happens for carbohydrate and fat for each of these different enzymes. That is the big role of digestive enzymes; without enzymes, we do not absorb our food.

The pancreas also has an endocrinal role; it produces and secretes two different endocrine hormones. One is called insulin, and the other is called glucagon. Insulin is needed for your cells to uptake the sugar that you absorb from your food. When you eat a carbohydrate, the enzymes will break it down to its base units into glucose. You absorb these units and then have peaks of glucose in your blood.

Your body cannot handle sugars peaks in your blood stream, so at that point insulin is secreted. It pushes the glucose from your blood stream into your cells. You need that insulin for the sugar to enter your cells, so that it can be used. When insulin is not doing its job of pushing glucose into your cells, glucose stays high in the blood stream and the condition soon leads to diabetes.

Alternatively, you have glucagon, another hormone secreted by the pancreas. This hormone does the opposite to insulin. For example, what happens if you do not eat for a while and your body needs some sugar for energy?

Since glucose is your main source of energy, your liver will pick up this situation, get the pancreas to secrete some glucagon hormone and this in turn then signals your cells to release their stored sugar.

That is how blood sugar is regulated in your body. It is done through the pancreas. Many overweight people have some form of poor blood-glucose regulation. A condition called metabolic syndrome is common and includes insulin resistance as one of its components.

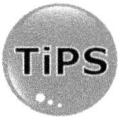

TiPS

1. Control and minimize the amount of splurging on simple sugars that are found in processed carbohydrates. They tend to be absorbed into your blood stream in great amounts, causing a peak of glucose that can overwhelm your insulin hormone. A huge dump of glucose into your blood is not ideal.

2. Instead, chose natural carbohydrates as they contain fiber. Fiber helps your insulin hormone as it slows down the absorption of glucose into your blood stream and does not cause an overwhelming glucose peak.

3. Increasing fiber in your diet helps you lose weight. Remember that processed carbohydrates are turned rapidly into simple sugars. They are absorbed into your blood stream causing a glucose peak. This overwhelms your pancreas because the hormone insulin has to sweep it up into the cells quickly. If the hormone insulin cannot sweep the glucose peak into the cells, fast enough it turns into fat.

4. Eat complex carbohydrates as they come from Mother Nature to avoid quick fat gain

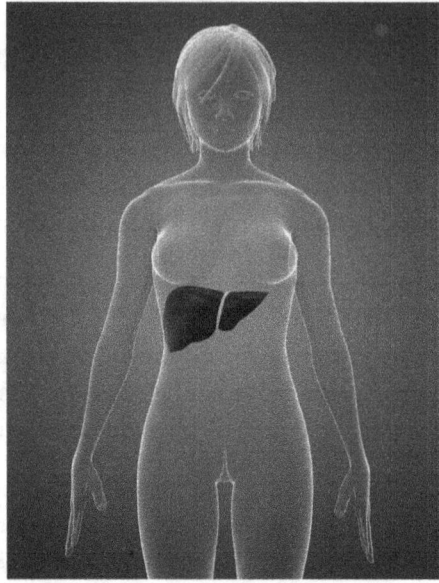

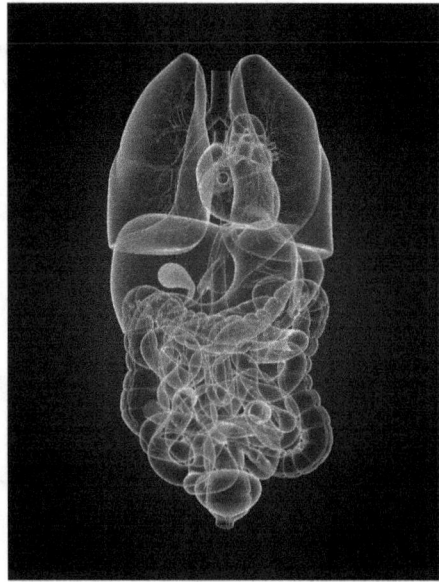

CHAPTER 8

Liver & Gall Bladder

Your liver is a wonderful organ. It sits on your upper abdomen and to the right of your stomach. Your liver produces bile, which is important for fat digestion, and the gall bladder and the liver work in combination. Your gall bladder is another interesting unit, which acts as a storage element, but unlike the rest of your internal organs, does not create anything.

Fat digestion is different from the digestion of carbohydrates and protein. Since oil and water do not mix, fat requires an emulsion factor to break it down, and that is what bile does. Bile aids in the digestion of fats, acting as an emulsifier to allow these enzymes to get into fat and break down the molecules into smaller amounts.

The bile your liver produces is stored in your gall bladder, where it is secreted as needed. Your liver is a gatekeeper and probably your hardest working organ. Amino acids, sugars and vitamins, all travel to the liver through what is known as the hepatic portal vein, and they are processed there. Some get stored, and some are sent out to the rest of your body. Your liver decides where and what things are stored, and what is eliminated. It is truly your best organ for health and weight loss.

Your liver's job is to detoxify and to look at everything in your body. It is checking out all the bi-products of the processes that happen there and making sure they are safe. It detoxifies toxins and drugs. Anything that is not safe for you is sent onto your urinary tract or colon and excreted out of your body. It is very important to keep your liver healthy.

To recap, your small intestine does most of the digestion and almost all the absorption, and it does it with the help of these accessory organs. Whatever is not absorbed moves onto your large intestine.

TiPS

1. Alcohol overloads your liver and prevents it from doing its job properly. Decrease your alcohol intake and stop if you can. You need a well-functioning liver to lose weight effectively.

2. Your liver makes bile that is important for fat metabolism. It is a good idea to look after your liver and support its bile making function for weight loss.

3. Cruciferous vegetables such as broccoli, cauliflower, and Brussels sprouts are supportive of the liver, as well as high in iron.

4. Vitamin B complex and milk thistle support liver. Take a multivitamin with a good dose of vitamin C and E daily.

5. Increase your consumption of green leafy vegetables

6. Minimize contact with toxins and unnecessary drug intakes.

7. Bitter tasting foods are good for the liver. You can buy a bottle of liver bitters at the local health shop and take a spoonful daily.

8. If your liver is sluggish, take a good liver herb tonic containing milk thistle, Dandelion and Globe Artichoke.

9. You liver needs to eliminate its detox products fast, so make sure you pass urine on time and not hold it in. This applies to pass your stools as well. When the urge is there, do not hold it in.

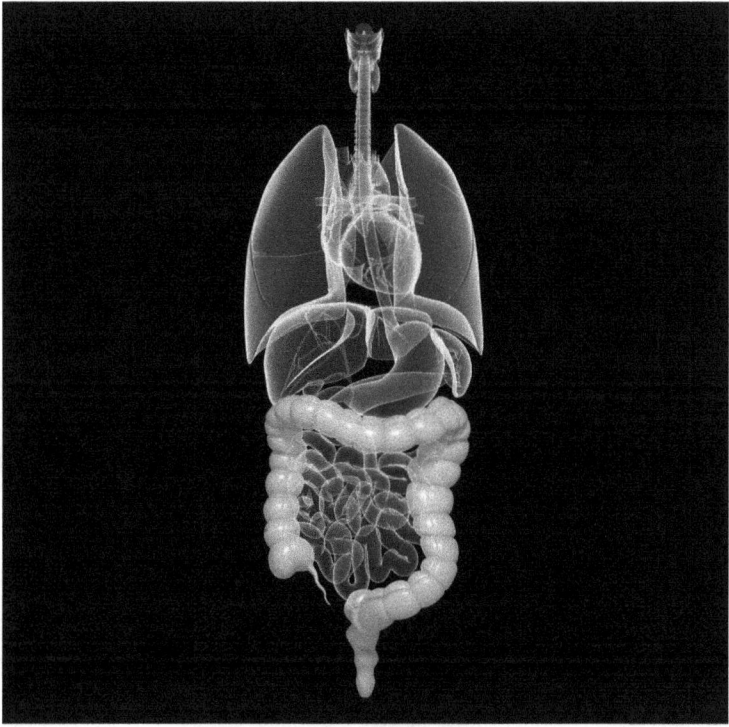

CHAPTER 9

Large Intestine

Your large intestine, otherwise known as the colon, is about 2-3 inches in diameter and only about 5 feet long. It receives watery waste containing undigested food from the small intestine. Water is also absorbed through the walls of your colon into the bloodstream, so you do not lose a lot of that water. You lose a bit in your feces, but anything that is in the large intestine typically gets re-absorbed by the body.

The liquid waste is transferred into a semi-solid waste that is your feces. This waste passes through your large intestine to the rectum and is expelled through your anus. When you move your bowels, it is eliminating waste out of your body.

Your fecal matter may stay in your colon for up to 24 hours. This is good for the growth of bacteria in your colon. There is a very large intestinal micro flora, about 300-500 species of bacteria, that reside in your colon. The bacteria in your gut is about 10 times greater than the human cells in your body, so you are primarily bacteria more than you are even human cells.

These bacteria help you break down the unabsorbed portion of your food, or fiber. You do not absorb fiber, and it is used to keep your large intestine healthy. Fiber is the nutrient for these bacteria, and it is how they flourish and promote good colon health. Bacteria also synthesize vitamin K. Most of the vitamin K in your body is created by the colon bacteria.

You can get vitamin K from some of your foods, mostly green leafy vegetables. It is re-absorbed through the lining of your large intestine and utilized by your body. When bacteria eat away the fiber, the result is CO_2 or gas in your colon.

This is why fiber causes gas, and all humans pass gas daily. Of course, some more than others but we all do. These bacteria are one of the ways you keep your large intestines healthy.

There are many things that damage these colon bacteria and many reasons why they get lost, like dehydration, antibiotics, poor diet and age. All of these can affect your digestive processes. It is important to keep that intestinal flora healthy, which helps to improve your digestion.

The food that you eat and how you digest it determines the rest of your health. It's often said, "you are what you eat" but it should be "you are what you digest and absorb."

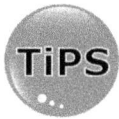

TiPS

1. Drink 2-3 liters of water to ensure a proper functioning of your colon.

2. Ensure regular movements of your bowel, every 1-2 days and empty it well in a relaxed manner.

3. Squat down to pass stools if possible as this is the best position to ensure smooth outflow.

4. Take your time to pass your motion; it is not a race. It is a very important part of the digestive system.

5. Take a good probiotic if you need one.

6. A good exercise routine helps the colon do its job well.

7. Eat less processed food.

8. Increase fiber intake if constipated, or to prevent constipation.

9. Minimize laxatives; instead, increase water and fiber in your diet.

10. If you are brave, have a colonic irrigation (this is not for everybody)

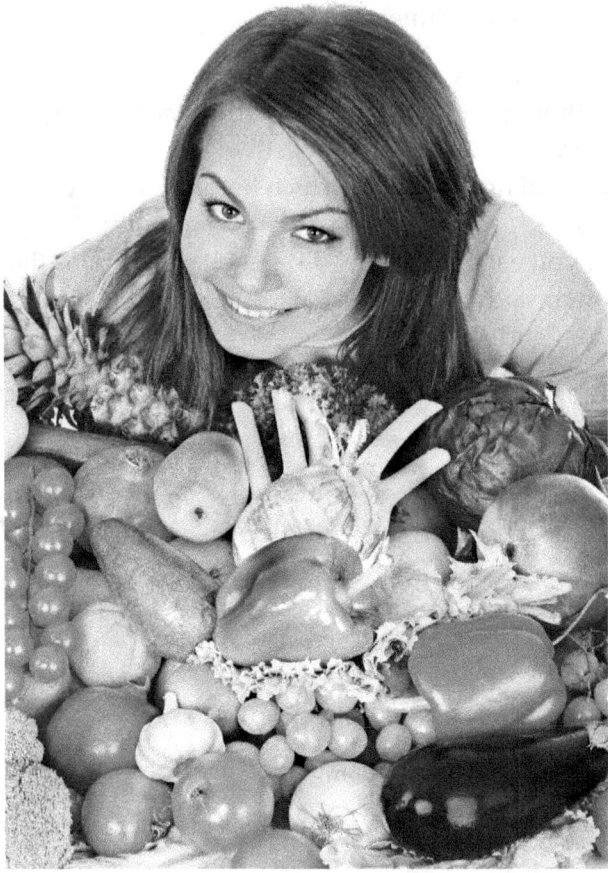

CHAPTER 10

You Are What You Eat

Good-quality organic food

Unfortunately, there is a problem with many of the foods that are readily available in the markets these days. Many people get fixated on the quantity of food and forget about the quality that is more important to your health.

The best quality food is the organic natural food; the way nature makes it. Go for natural organic as much as you can. It may appear more costly, but the quality is unbeatable. You eat less of the organic food because your body absorbs more nutrition from it. Therefore, it ends up costing about the same as the mass-produced food in the supermarket.

For those who say the local health shop is too expensive, try the farmer's market. It is cheaper than the organic shop and still good for you. Many of them start early in the morning, 7:30 until noon. Therefore, it requires that you get up early on a Saturday to stock up on organically grown healthy foods. These local farmers need your support for their business. There is no excuse for this one. Their prices are affordable and comparable to the supermarket prices. There are plenty of reasons why you should eat organically grown natural foods from Mother Nature. Price argument is not valid!

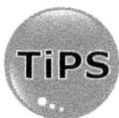

TiPS

1. Stock up on organic food from your local farmer shop. It is affordable, locally grown organic food, and they need your support. Your body will thank you for it.

2. Quality of food is better than quantity.

3. You consume less of the organic quality food since your body absorbs more nutrition from them.

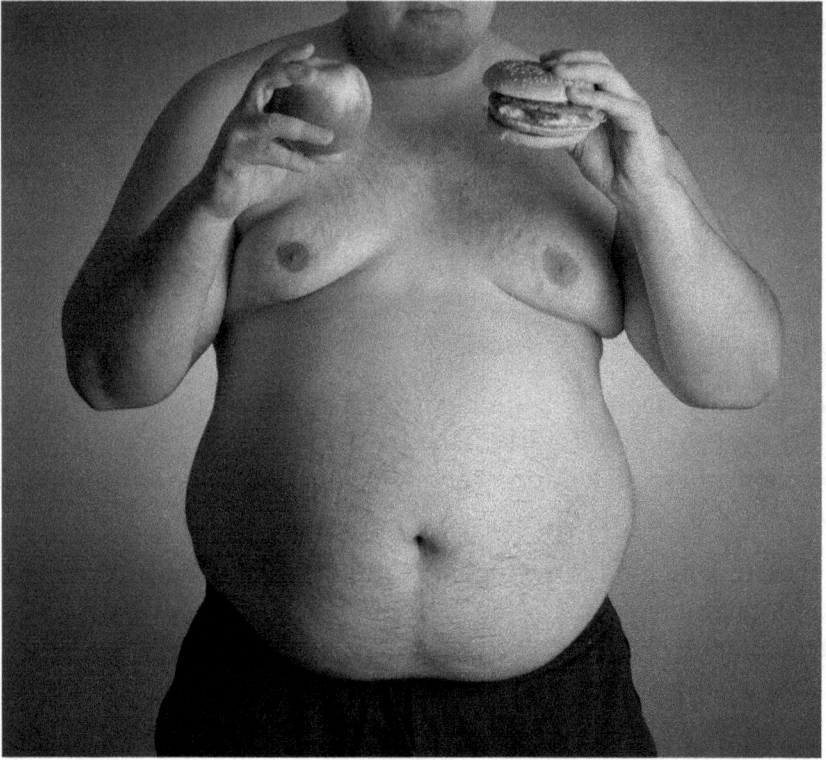

CHAPTER 11

How To Tell True Hunger

There are many forms of hunger

There is hunger and there is being hungry. Many people do not know what it truly feels like to be hungry. Over-hunger can lead to over-eating and binging; therefore, to weight gain. Too many people live on liquid diets like cups of coffees, cokes, sweetened drinks, and Frappuccino.

The more liquids they consume, the less likely they are to know whether they are hungry or not. Liquid diets bypass the chewing of food that is important in digestion. By chewing their food, they slow down their digestion.

People are drinking their food because they are in such a hurry, they are moving along so quickly. If people do not acknowledge that they are hungry, they will go long periods without eating. Then they are ravenous and when this happens, they tend to binge eat. In addition, they do not make very good choices.

There are a few kinds of hunger to be aware of. There is taste hunger. This is when you eat because it sounds good or because the occasion calls for it. For people who are healthy eaters, this is no problem. For example, you might go to an event, and Grandma has made her special cream puffs. You are going to eat them whether you are hungry or not, whether you need them or not. It is not a matter of being hungry. This kind of eating is appropriate.

There is also practical hunger. You might be planning and eating even though you are not hungry. You might be going to the movies, and although you are not hungry at 5 o'clock, you are not going to get another chance to eat until 10 o'clock. Have a light snack, a salad or something that keeps you satisfied. If you do not do this, you could end up overeating or binging.

Lastly, there is emotional hunger, or stress eating. This is where cravings come into play and where it requires a little more work. You eat trying to clench your uncomfortable feelings. This is the hunger you feel when you are trying not to be bored, lonely or angry.

This is the time when you keep opening the fridge and stand there deciding what you are craving. You know that there is an uncomfortable feeling, and it is out of control. This feeling is identical to over-eating and whether it is triggered emotionally or biologically, it is going to feel the same. It feels like you are hungry even though you might have eaten. You just keep taking trips to the kitchen to eat more.

Then there is the real and true hunger for food. You feel different when you are truly hungry. There is a growling feeling in your stomach, and you feel a bit light headed. It has a physical feeling to it.

I recommend eating only when you are truly hungry. Eat three big meals with smaller snacks in between. Do not go any longer than five hours without eating. Check yourself to notice your hunger levels. Ask yourself, when was the last time you ate and how you are feeling physically?

These are good things to do when you are thinking about healthy eating. Do not underestimate the value of slowing down to check whether your hunger is real or a craving for something else.

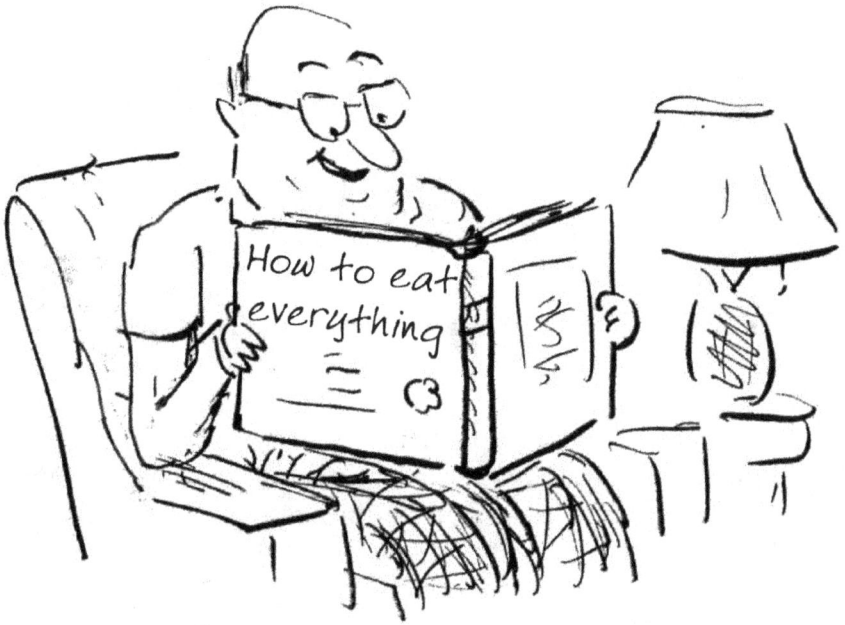

CHAPTER 12

How To Eat Your Food

Eating is something you do unconsciously. Today people do not the take time to appreciate their meal times. My guess is that they are too busy on mobile phones, computers, Facebook or watching soap operas. There are too many things occupying their time these days and this does not encourage good digestion. Digestion is part of the parasympathetic nervous system that is dominant during rest and relaxation. You must start paying more attention to your digestion. Eat in peace and tranquility, give yourself time to eat and do not share your meal times with your daily troubles. Keep your mind positive at meal times to encourage better digestion. Switch off the TV while eating as it distracts from proper chewing and enjoyment of your food.

It is not helpful to your digestion to gobble down a large meal in front of the TV. It is detrimental to your waistline, because you do not control how much food is passing through your lips. You end up eating beyond your satiation point because you are not conscious enough to listen to your brain's signals. You are too involved with what is on the TV and eat on autopilot. You gobble down a large packet of chips and then wonder how you did it. All you recall is opening the packet and wanting to eat just a little and now the whole bag is empty.

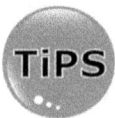

TiPS

1. Eat in a peaceful place.

2. Do not eat in front of the TV. You become too involved in the TV and end up eating much more than needed.

3. Have positive thoughts while eating and forget about your troubles for a bit. Allow your mind to be peaceful.

4. Be conscious of every mouthful to enjoy the taste and flavor.

5. Say a prayer of gratitude before and after the meal.

6. Sit down to eat, do not stand or move around.

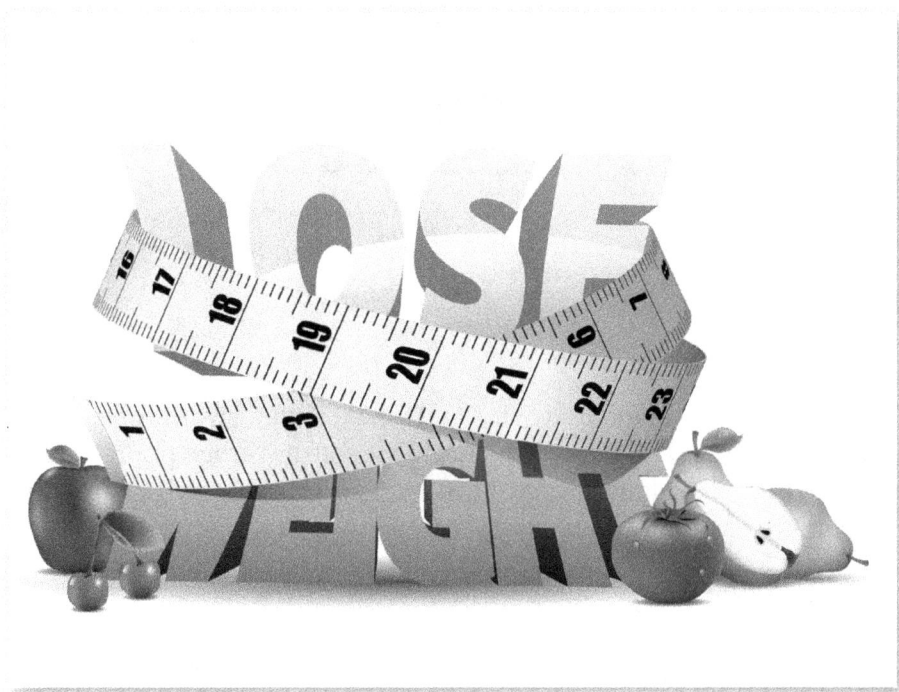

CHAPTER 13

Eating For
Weight-Loss Success

Have you ever wondered why you eat? Obviously, you eat when you are hungry. More significantly, you have been taught how and when to eat. Many of you have learned to eat three meals a day regardless of whether you are hungry or not. As children, you were forced to finish your meal. Your body was being stuffed to above its capacity.

As an adult, that program has solidified in your mind and runs the show. I find it strange when parents complain that teenagers are fat. It is parents who teach their children how to eat and how to stuff their faces, whether they wanted to clean their plates or not.

The mind and body have a relationship in which they interchange commands and information. When it comes to food, your mind decides what the rules to eating are. Your mind gives that command that you must eat three times a day and wipe your plate clean. Otherwise, you are ungrateful and wasteful since there are kids starving in Africa.

Not only do you inherit the idea of how much and how often to eat; you are implanted with guilt from the environment you grew up in. When you look at people from distinct backgrounds, you notice that their food portions are different. You may think you eat too much, but when you go to other countries, you see that they may consume more than you do.

Different cultures have different amounts of what is healthy for them to consume. In my health programs, I do not focus on how much you eat but *what* you eat. I have clients all over the world from different cultures and backgrounds. I don't follow any set standard.

The purpose of food is to provide nutrients for calories, energy, and maintenance, and to repair of your body. Nutrients are also needed for growth, metabolism, and for all your body functions. Macro means large, and macronutrients are those needed in the largest amounts by your body.

These macronutrients are carbohydrates, proteins and fats. This is opposed to the micronutrients, which are vitamins and minerals that play a role in your wellness.

While each of these macronutrients provides calories, the amount of calories they provide varies. Proteins and carbohydrates both provide 4 calories per gram. Fats provide a lot more. They provide 9 calories per gram.

Besides carbohydrates, proteins and fats, there is another substance that you take in that provides calories. It is alcohol that provides 7 calories per gram; it is closer in caloric level to fat. However, it is not considered a macronutrient because you do not need it for your survival.

Let us look at the macronutrients, carbohydrates, proteins, and fats.

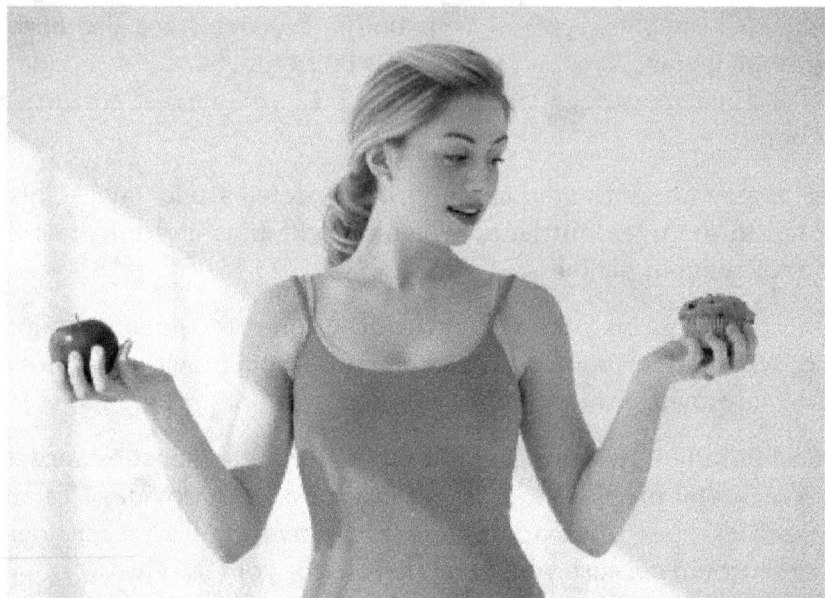

CHAPTER 14

Eating Carbohydrates:
The Good Vs. The Bad Carbs

Carbohydrates, or carbs, are foods that are abundant in nature. This is what you eat the most, and what your body requires more than anything else does because they provide the primary source of energy for your body. On average, you will need about 50% to 60% of your daily total caloric intake to come from carbohydrates, and that is a lot of carbs.

The big question is not about how much you take in, but the *quality* of carbohydrate you are eating. The carb question is the most common question that I am asked.

The solution to this question is never to starve your body of its much-needed carbs, but invest in good-quality carbs that actually help you lose weight.

No matter what form of carbohydrate you take in, your body will convert it to its simplest form, glucose, which is where the energy comes from. When your body does not need the energy, the glucose produces; you store it in your cells, muscles and liver as glycogen to be used later. Your body needs energy to survive, and carbs provide it. Carbohydrates are also needed for our intestinal health, which is waste elimination in the colon.

Natural carbohydrates do not peak your sugars when they are absorbed into your blood stream. Therefore, they do not trigger a lot of insulin hormone reactions.

Poor-quality carbs spike your blood sugars when they are absorbed into your blood stream, causing massive amounts of the hormone insulin to be released, in order to push glucose into your blood. This is a problem because the excess processed carbs in the blood stream is turned into fat stores quickly.

This is why the best carbs to eat are the natural complex carbs that have natural fiber. These fibers slow down absorption into the blood stream triggering a slower release of insulin. This way insulin takes its time pushing the glucose into your cells, and if you eat good, complex carbs, you will have more energy available and will not gain weight too quickly as compared to the processed carbs.

I am not telling you to eat fewer carbs because that would starve your body of its primary needed nutrient and energy source. Instead, eat less of the processed carbs that are found in junk foods and spike your blood sugars, and choose things that have fiber and are absorbed slowly into the blood stream.

They will keep you well energized throughout the day by using the energy instead of the hormone insulin storing it as fat. Eat more rather than less, as carbohydrates are your primary energy source for the body.

Carbohydrates are found in plant foods such as fruit, vegetables, grains, legumes, nuts and seeds. The exception is lactose, which is the sugar found in milk. Often people cannot digest lactose, or as they age, many people will become lactose intolerant.

All your body tissues and cells can use glucose for energy, and it is the sole source of the brain. Carbohydrates are also needed for your central nervous system that includes your kidneys, brain and the muscles of your heart to function properly.

Refining carbohydrates is an unnatural process designed to make them look more appealing when they are sold. A processed carb undergoes refining to remove the coarse parts of the original form. For example, look at a grain of brown rice versus a grain of white rice.

Brown rice is the natural whole grain containing two layers on the outside. One layer is called the bran and the other layer is the germ. They both contain fiber, B vitamins, trace minerals, vitamin E and other vital nutrients. On the other hand, the white starchy center of the rice grain is called the endosperm, which is what we are familiar with when we think of white rice.

This is what is left when the outer nutritious layers are removed from brown rice, and when you eat this processed rice, all you are consuming is that starchy carb center, which is just a ball of sugar chains.

The reason why it is important to consume things in their completely natural form is because otherwise, we lose many of the foods nutrients. It is an acquired taste to eat brown rice, but you will get used to it. You will notice how much more energy you have during the day and how regular your bowel motions become. The fiber in the natural whole grains helps digestion.

We know that diet is a major problem in many countries. Most people consume carbohydrates in the form of refined unnatural foods. This can lead to an overload of sugars in their system. It also increases the risks of obesity, diabetes or insulin resistance, heart disease, and high cholesterol and triglycerides. Even other diseases like cancer and autoimmune disorders can be connected to high intakes of refined unnatural carbohydrates.

The next way we classify carbohydrates is as simple and complex. Good carbs or "complex carbs" are the choice foods while "simple carbs" like white rice are bad.

One of the most common simple sugars is fruit. Sugars are made up of sugar molecules linked together. Simple sugars are one sugar or two molecules linked together. Simple sugars that are found in nature are glucose, fructose (sugar found in fruit and honey), GA lactose, di-saccharides (maltose, sucrose – table sugar), sugar beets, sugar cane, maple syrup and lactose (which is the sugar found in milk).

All these types of sugar are either simple sugars of monosaccharaides, or simple sugars of di-saccharides. Due to their simple molecular structure, they are typically digested more easily and quickly. They do not need to be broken down that much to be converted into glucose form or the blood sugar that we need.

When you have a simple unrefined or whole sugar, such as an apple, it will be absorbed slower than a piece of candy that is also made up of simple sugar. The apple peel contains fiber that will slow down your digestion and absorption, whereas the sugar in the candy does not have any fiber to help slow things down. As well as fiber, there are many good nutrients in the apple. Therefore, it is important to consume that type of simple sugars.

Unrefined complex carbohydrates are fibers, starches or what is commonly known as polysaccharides (many molecules linked together). We store polysaccharides in our body as glycogen. Plants store sugar in the form of starch. Among many starchy foods are potatoes, cereals, whole grains, corn and peas. Foods that contain a lot of fiber, which are also complex carbohydrates include legumes, broccoli, cauliflower, spinach and other leafy greens.

Fiber is an important carbohydrate for your health as it aids digestion. There are two different types of fiber, soluble fiber and insoluble fiber. Soluble fiber is soluble in water so as it goes through your body it absorbs water. That water is added to your stool, so it increases the bulk and the weight of your feces. You can find soluble fiber in oats, the inside of fruits, beans and some seaweed.

Insoluble fiber is insoluble in water, which means that it does not absorb water as it is going through your system. This means it goes through quickly, which increases the speed at which your stool moves through your body. Insoluble fiber is in wheat, rye and most of our vegetables.

Many natural foods contain both soluble and insoluble fiber. The peel of an apple will be mostly insoluble, whereas the inside part will be soluble fiber. Oatmeal will swell and get somewhat gelatinous when you add water because it is soluble in water.

When oatmeal soaks up water, it adds bulk to our stools. However, you can add all the water you want to cream of wheat, but the grains will not get any bigger meaning the grains are *insoluble*.

When you read a packaged food label, you see 'dietary fiber'. Dietary fiber contains both soluble and insoluble fiber because they are both needed by the body. We need to have a stool that has weight and bulk so that it moves out of the body quickly.

Fiber is needed to promote a healthy gut function because it helps facilitate elimination. You can think of fiber as a type of scrub brush for our intestines. Fiber also promotes a healthy gut flora. Your colon has both good and bad bacteria in it. You want to have good rather than bad bacteria. It also reduces the risk of colon cancer because it keeps your colon from becoming constipated, and therefore, you can eliminate feces from your body.

Soluble fiber also reduces cholesterol. Often you will see a red heart symbol on a box of oatmeal. That is because it has been shown that soluble fiber not only binds with water, it can also bind with cholesterol and keep that cholesterol from being absorbed. It can help eliminate a lot of cholesterol from your body.

Fiber helps maintain a healthy weight. When you consume foods that have a lot of fiber, they keep you feeling fuller longer. It slows down your digestion and because fiber absorbs water, it adds bulk to your stomach and digestive tract. You end up eating less of the foods that have a lot of fiber because you get full quicker, and you stay full longer. That means you eat less often.

Diets that are low in fiber have been shown to lead to an increased risk of constipation, hemorrhoids, diverticulosis, obesity and diabetes, and increase the risk for colon cancer.

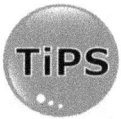

TiPS

1. About 25-35 grams per day is the usual recommendation. I think it is more important to be upwards of 40 grams per day. This can be done if you are consuming fruits, vegetables and whole-grain carbohydrate foods regularly.

2. Avoid refined foods and have fruits and vegetables with all your meals.

3. Eat 50%-60% natural carbohydrates.

4. Remember your brain uses carbohydrates for energy, so be careful when restricting your carbs.

5. Decrease processed carbs and increase natural carbs, as they are your primary source of energy in the body.

6. Eat brown color versions of carbs as they still contain their nutritious values. White bleached color carbs have been stripped of their natural fibers and nutrition.

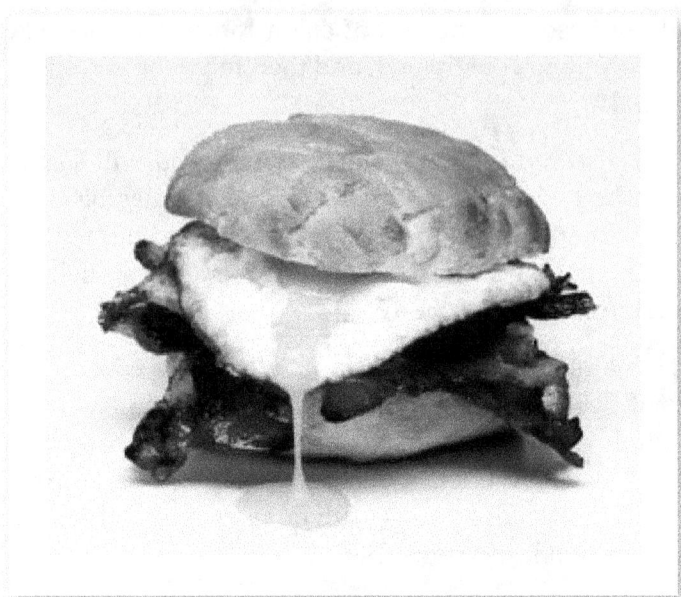

CHAPTER 15

Eating Fats:
The Good, The Bad & The Ugly

Fats are the most hated nutrient in the world and have received bad press for a long time. It is time to change that because it has been exaggerated long enough. Your body needs fat. Every cell in your body has a cell membrane that contains fat molecules. Some fats are essential for your survival.

Usually, about 20-30% of our daily calories should come from healthy fat. Fats are needed for normal growth and development. Your body uses fat for energy as well. Fat is the second form of energy fuel the body uses after glucose. The body also uses fat to protect its internal organs.

Fat plays two major roles, organ protection and energy storage, and it protects you more than you know. You need fat to absorb fat-soluble vitamins such as vitamins A, D, E and K, as well as providing cushioning for your organs from trauma or change of internal environment. In foods, it provides that yummy taste, consistency and stability. Fat is stored in outer-post tissue, under the skin and around the organs; because of this, it insulates the body, and protects it from shocks. Fat in the form of cholesterol is also used to produce some hormones in the body, like testosterone.

You can find fat in many delicious and different food sources. It is found in animal products like meat, poultry and milk products, as well as fish and some plant-based sources like seeds, nuts and some grains.

There are three different types of fats: saturated fats, unsaturated fats and trans-fats. In saturated fats, all the carbon atoms are saturated with hydrogen molecules. They are solid at room temperature and are found mostly in animal foods.

Coconut oil is also solid at room temperature and contains a type of saturated fat. It is healthier than the animal saturated fats and more stable at high temperatures.

Unsaturated fats have only some of the carbon molecules attached to the hydrogen molecules, and there are two kinds of unsaturated fats.

One is mono-unsaturated fats that are primarily found in olive oil, peanut oil and canola. The other is poly-unsaturated fats that are in fish oil, corn oil and soya bean oil. Essential fatty acids are poly-unsaturated and are called Omega-3 and Omega-6 fatty acids. They are essential because your body cannot make its own supply.

Therefore, you need to get them into your diet. Few people consume enough Omega-3 essential oils as they are found in very specific foods such as walnuts, flax seeds and in fatty fish like salmon. Omega-6 fatty acid is also available in foods such as nuts, corn, sunflower and some oils.

Trans fats are unsaturated fats that have been saturated with hydrogen. These become softer at room temperature and are spreadable like butter. They are made by adding hydrogen to oil so that no more carbon molecules can attach to the hydrogen.

This process solidifies the oil and makes it softer than butter. When you read a food label, you will often see the term hydrogenated oil. Hydrogenated corn oil and hydrogenated soy oil are examples. The term hydrogenated means its trans-fat. It is a more stable fat that can be cooked at a higher temperature. It also last longer on the shelf (increased shelf life) which is why many food companies use it.

However, this is the kind of fat you need to be careful of because it raises your bad cholesterol levels, increases the risk for heart disease and is now thought to be worse than saturated fat in the body.

Saturated fats as well as trans-fats have been shown to increase the risk of heart disease, heart cholesterol levels and hardening of your arteries. Therefore, when you are looking at food labels watch out for anything that says partially hydrogenated.

When you are reading labels, it is important to read the ingredient list, not just the numbers or percentages. In the ingredient list, if you see the word partially hydrogenated or hydrogenated it is something to avoid if getting healthy is your goal.

Even though unsaturated fats are healthy for your body and saturated and trans-fatty acids are not, over consumption of any kind of fat can lead to health problems. Some of these are obesity, cardiovascular disease, elevated cholesterol and triglycerides, cancer and fatty liver disease.

The point is that you can eat too much olive oil. You do want to get mono-unsaturated and poly-unsaturated fats in your diet. That means both the essential fats like the Omega-3 and mono-unsaturated like olive oil because those fats provide many good health benefits, if consumed in moderation.

Olive oil is actually thought to lower your bad cholesterol and keep your good cholesterol high, the way we want it to be. It also protects your heart. This can happen only in moderate amounts.

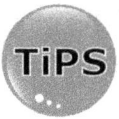

TiPS

1. You need fats in your diet to maintain your healthy body. Depriving your body is unhealthy and leads to ill health.

2. Good fats are filling and add flavor to foods.

3. Do not over-consume any forms of fats; just eat enough of them to be healthy.

4. You need to take supplements of Omega-3 as they are essential and your body does not produce them. Since they are found in very few foods, they may not be on your list of frequently eaten foods.

5. Read product labels carefully to see which type of fats have been used in the product.

6. Get more of the mono-unsaturated oil and poly-unsaturated fats in your diet, and minimize the trans-fats and hydrogenated fats.

7. Minimize the consumption of animal fats and saturated fats.

8. Do not be afraid of fats, they protect your vital organs, and that is a good thing.

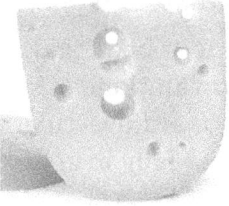

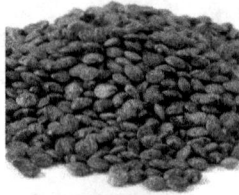

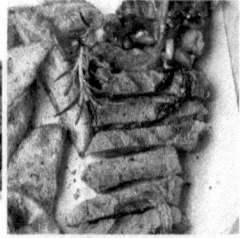

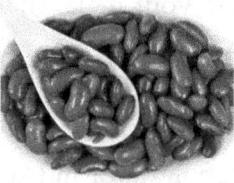

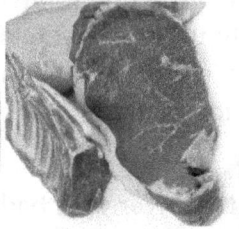

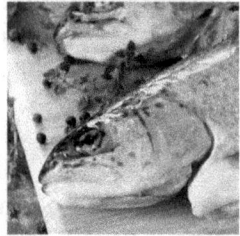

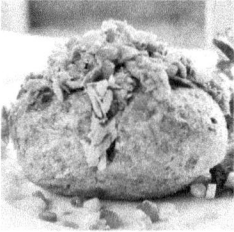

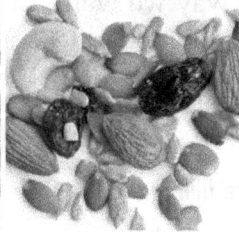

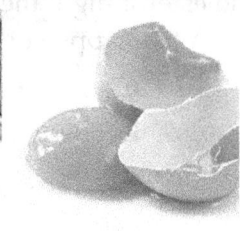

CHAPTER 16

Eating Proteins:
The Structure Re-Builder

The chemical structures of protein are amino acids, all strung together. Many foods contain some proteins. Protein is needed for growth, especially during children's younger years, and for pregnant women. It is needed for tissue repair, immune function and making essential hormones and enzymes. It regulates our fluid and pH balance.

Protein is also needed for building collagen that holds your cells together and provides the framework for your bones and teeth. Protein can also provide energy when carbohydrates and fats are not available or are limited.

The best thing about protein is that it preserves lean muscle mass. Eating too much protein does not build muscle. You cannot sit around eating protein and expect your muscles to get bigger. This is the high-protein diet myth that many people buy into and can actually end up being very bad for you. The only way to build larger muscles is to work them, with such exercises as weight lifting and resistance training.

To build muscle, you have to work out and challenge the muscles to tone them up. While doing that, you need to consume protein to maintain the building processes, but you cannot eat your way to sexy lean muscles. You have to do the work too.

There are two major sources of protein, plant-based protein and animal protein. Plant proteins provide the added benefits of fiber and can provide some iron, zinc and calcium. In addition to that, they provide certain chemicals and unsaturated fats.

Unfortunately, a plant-based protein diet does not provide vitamin B12. All the other B vitamins are found both in plant and animal tissues. Iron from plant foods is not easily absorbed. If you have an iron deficiency, (anemia) it can be very difficult to get your iron up through a plant-based diet alone.

Iron is needed for energy levels as it forms part of the red blood cells that transport oxygen. Plant proteins are found in nuts, beans, legumes, soy, and even some whole grains.

Animal proteins are from meats, poultry, any animal flesh, dairy products and egg products. Animal proteins provide B vitamins, iron, zinc and calcium. However, they have no fiber and are often high in cholesterol and unsaturated fat.

Our needs from protein vary from person to person. In general, we need anywhere from 10% to 15% protein in our daily diet. Most people get enough protein and when the high-protein diet craze was popular, people were getting too much protein.

Your body does not store excessive amino acids, so you are not really storing excessive protein. When you take in too much protein, it is converted to fatty acids. This can lead to weight gain as the fatty acids are stored as fat. The body uses up as much of the protein as it can to repair and rebuild other compounds. Just remember that you do not have the storage capacity for it as you do for carbohydrates or fat.

There are some dangers to the high-protein diets. Protein breakdown is a bi-product called urea, and it must be eliminated, which increases water loss. Furthermore, too much protein can cause excretion of calcium in the urine and can lead to kidney stones and bone loss.

There is some indication that long-term excessive protein intake can lead to kidney and liver damage. A typical high-protein diet is low in fruit and vegetables, low in fiber and high in cholesterol and saturated fats. Not only can this diet cause damage to your body, but also it will lack many other needed nutrients.

TiPS

1. Eat protein at every meal.

2. The first 2-3 mouthfuls should be proteins, since this helps you not to over eat. You can never pig out on proteins as much as you can on processed carbs. Try it at home and see what I mean.

3. Get lean meat.

4. Get free range or organic eggs.

5. Use high-quality protein for your body because it repairs your structures.

6. Strength training is important in muscle building, and proteins help support the process.

7. Do not overeat proteins because they will affect your kidneys.

8. You do not have room to store extra protein, and it will eventually turn to fat.

9. Drink lots of water if you increase your protein intake.

   Vegetarian protein intake needs to be supplemented by vitamin B12, as it is not found in plant protein.

7 MOST ALKALINE FOODS

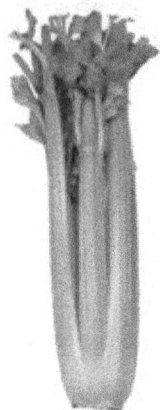

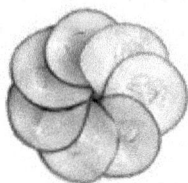

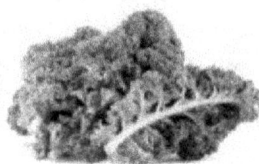

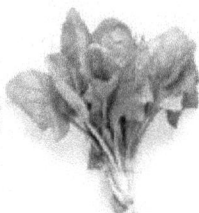

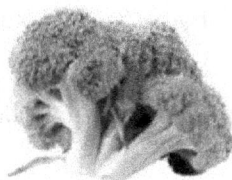

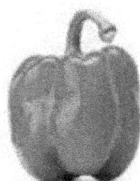

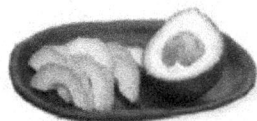

CHAPTER 17

Eating Alkaline Foods

The way that you digest food influences the acid-based balance in your body. The food that you eat shifts your PH either into acidity or into alkalinity. The digestive system can be affected by stress patterns, negative emotions and low immunity, which push the body towards a more acid PH.

All the food you eat leaves an ash residue after metabolism that is either alkaline or acid. This depends on the mineral composition of the foods, and the way that your body digests them. Foods are classified according to their effect at the end of your digestive and metabolic processes. They are either neutral; acidic-forming or alkaline-forming (see charts of alkaline-acid foods lists).

...ALKALINE FOODS...	...ACIDIC FOODS...
ALKALIZING VEGETABLES	**ACIDIFYING VEGETABLES**
Alfalfa	Corn
Barley Grass	Lentils
Beet Greens	Olives
Beets	Winter Squash
Broccoli	
Cabbage	**ACIDIFYING FRUITS**
Carrot	Blueberries
Cauliflower	Canned or Glazed Fruits
Celery	Cranberries
Chard Greens	Currants
Chlorella	Plums**
Collard Greens	Prunes**
Cucumber	
Dandelions	**ACIDIFYING GRAINS, GRAIN PRODUCTS**
Dulce	Amaranth
Edible Flowers	Barley
Eggplant	Bran, oat
Fermented Veggies	Bran, wheat
Garlic	Bread
Green Beans	Corn
Green Peas	Cornstarch
Kale	Crackers, soda
Kohlrabi	Flour, wheat
Lettuce	Flour, white
Mushrooms	Hemp Seed Flour
Mustard Greens	Kamut
Nightshade Veggies	Macaroni
Onions	Noodles
Parsnips (high glycemic)	Oatmeal
Peas	Oats (rolled)
Peppers	Quinoa
Pumpkin	Rice (all)

...ALKALINE FOODS...	...ACIDIC FOODS...
Radishes	Rice Cakes
Rutabaga	Rye
Sea Veggies	Spaghetti
Spinach, green	Spelt
Spirulina	Wheat Germ
Sprouts	Wheat
Sweet Potatoes	
Tomatoes	**ACIDIFYING BEANS & LEGUMES**
Watercress	Almond Milk
Wheat Grass	Black Beans
Wild Greens	Chick Peas
	Green Peas
ALKALIZING ORIENTAL	Kidney Beans
VEGETABLES	
Daikon	Lentils
Dandelion Root	Pinto Beans
Kombu	Red Beans
Maitake	Rice Milk
Nori	Soy Beans
Reishi	Soy Milk
Shitake	White Beans
Umeboshi	
Wakame	**ACIDIFYING DAIRY**
	Butter
ALKALIZING FRUITS	Cheese
Apple	Cheese, Processed
Apricot	Ice Cream
Avocado	Ice Milk
Banana (high glycemic)	
Berries	**ACIDIFYING NUTS & BUTTERS**
Blackberries	Cashews
Cantaloupe	Legumes
Cherries, sour	Peanut Butter

...ALKALINE FOODS...	...ACIDIC FOODS...
Coconut, fresh	Peanuts
Currants	Pecans
Dates, dried	Tahini
Figs, dried	Walnuts
Grapes	
Grapefruit	ACIDIFYING ANIMAL PROTEIN
Honeydew Melon	Bacon
Lemon	Beef
Lime	Carp
Muskmelons	Clams
Nectarine	Cod
Orange	Corned Beef
Peach	Fish
Pear	Haddock
Pineapple	Lamb
Raisins	Lobster
Raspberries	Mussels
Rhubarb	Organ Meats
Strawberries	Oyster
Tangerine	Pike
Tomato	Pork
Tropical Fruits	Rabbit
Umeboshi Plums	Salmon
Watermelon	Sardines
	Sausage
ALKALIZING PROTEIN	Scallops
Almonds	Shellfish
Chestnuts	Shrimp
Millet	Tuna
Tempeh (fermented)	Turkey
Tofu (fermented)	Veal
Whey Protein Powder	Venison

...ALKALINE FOODS...	...ACIDIC FOODS...
ALKALIZING SWEETENERS	ACIDIFYING FATS & OILS
Stevia	Avacado Oil
	Butter
ALKALIZING SPICES & SEASONINGS	Canola Oil
Chili Pepper	Corn Oil
Cinnamon	Flax Oil
Curry	Hemp Seed Oil
Ginger	Lard
Herbs (all)	Olive Oil
Miso	Safflower Oil
Mustard	Sesame Oil
Sea Salt	Sunflower Oil
Tamari	
	ACIDIFYING SWEETENERS
ALKALIZING OTHER	Carob
Alkaline Antioxidant Water	Corn Syrup
Apple Cider Vinegar	Sugar
Bee Pollen	
Fresh Fruit Juice	ACIDIFYING ALCOHOL
Green Juices	Beer
Lecithin Granules	Hard Liquor
Mineral Water	Spirits
Molasses, blackstrap	Wine
Probiotic Cultures	
Soured Dairy Products	ACIDIFYING OTHER FOODS
Veggie Juices	Catsup
	Cocoa
ALKALIZING MINERALS	Coffee
Calcium: pH 12	Mustard
Cesium: pH 14	Pepper
Magnesium: pH 9	Soft Drinks
Potassium: pH 14	Vinegar
Sodium: pH 14	

...ALKALINE FOODS...	...ACIDIC FOODS...
Although it might seem that citrus fruits would have an acidifying effect on the body, the citric acid they contain actually has an alkalinizing effect in the system.	**ACIDIFYING DRUGS & CHEMICALS** Aspirin Chemicals Drugs, Medicinal Drugs, Psychedelic Herbicides Pesticides Tobacco
Note that a food's acid or alkaline forming tendency in the body has nothing to do with the actual pH of the food itself. For example, lemons are very acidic, however the end products they produce after digestion and assimilation are very alkaline so, lemons are alkaline forming in the body. Likewise, meat will test alkaline before digestion, but it leaves very acidic residue in the body so, like nearly all animal products, meat is very acid forming.	**ACIDIFYING JUNK FOOD** Beer: pH 2.5 Coca-Cola: pH 2 Coffee: pH 4

A body that has an excessive acid ash will hang on to fat for protection. The presence of acidity in your blood stream gives your body a reason for storing fat that will supersede your wish to lose weight. It is the time when you go out of your way to go to the gym, to work out and to eat right, but you do not see the kilos drop. Sometime people even gain weight while dieting because they have too much acid in their system. If you are exercising beyond your capacity and not breathing well during the exercise, you are producing more acid in your body in the form of lactic acid. For example, you find your body cannot go on anymore, and yet you keep pushing and pushing because you have to fit onto that size 8 bikini in two months. You are creating more and more acid that is working against you rather than for you. Not to mention the stress you are putting your body under. This stress is activating your sympathetic nervous system that uses glucose and protein for energy and hardly ever touches the fat you want to lose.

Too much acid in your body leads to erosion. Look at some people's teeth and see the effect of acid erosion. When you change your diet to a more alkaline diet, your teeth become stronger and healthier.

Too much acid similarly leads to bone erosion. Your body desperately needs to neutralize the acid in your blood levels by eroding calcium and magnesium from your bones. Your bones become weaker and weaker.

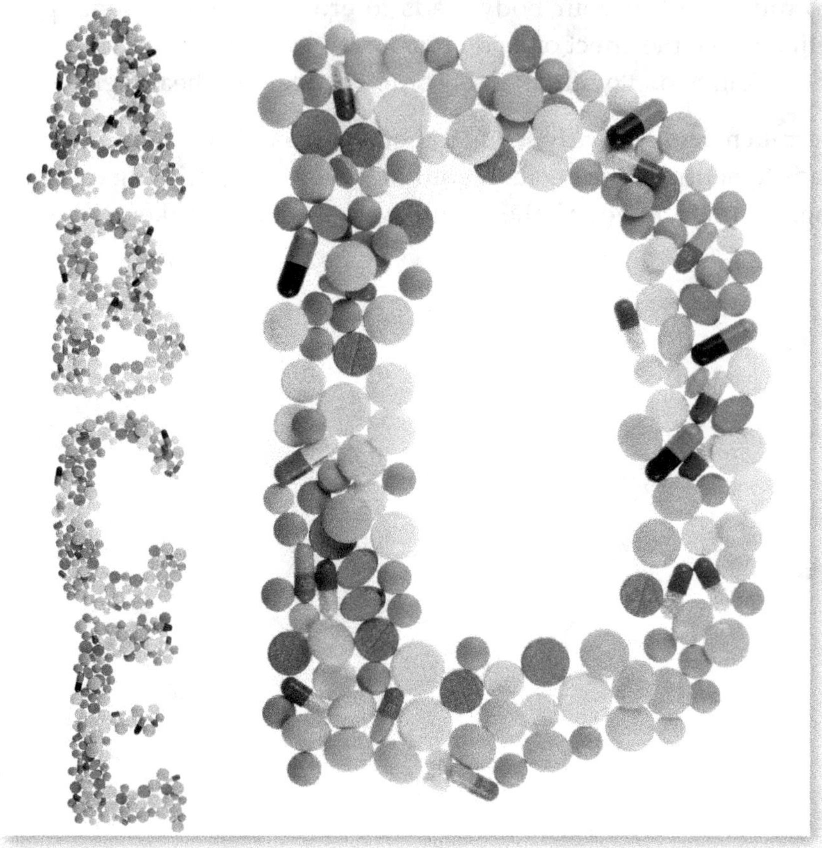

CHAPTER 18

Healthy Vitamins For
Your Body (Micro-Nutrients)

The human body needs multiple vitamins; they perform different functions to keep us healthy. However, they are needed in smaller amounts and are called micronutrients, as compared to macronutrients such as carbohydrates and proteins. We get the vitamins from our healthy food intake. Their functions are specialized. Vitamins are classified as either water-soluble or fat soluble, meaning they need either water or fat to be digested and absorbed into your body.

We have nine different water-soluble vitamins that include:

- Vitamin C
- Eight B Vitamins
  - Thiamine
  - Riboflavin
  - Niacin
  - Pantothenic Acid
  - Pyridoxine
  - Cyanocobalamin
  - Biotin
  - Folic Acid

There are also four fat-soluble vitamins:

- A
- D
- E
- K

Minerals are classified as either trace or major.   Our major minerals include:

- Calcium
- Phosphorous
- Potassium
- Sodium
- Chloride
- Magnesium
- Sulfur

Our trace minerals include:

- Iron
- Iodine
- Zinc
- Chromium
- Selenium
- Fluoride
- Molybdenum
- Copper
- Manganese

Vitamins are organic compounds; this means they can contain carbon in their structure and are essential for life. Vitamins are vulnerable to heat and light. This means that food preparation, processing, and storage are important to preserve them in our food.

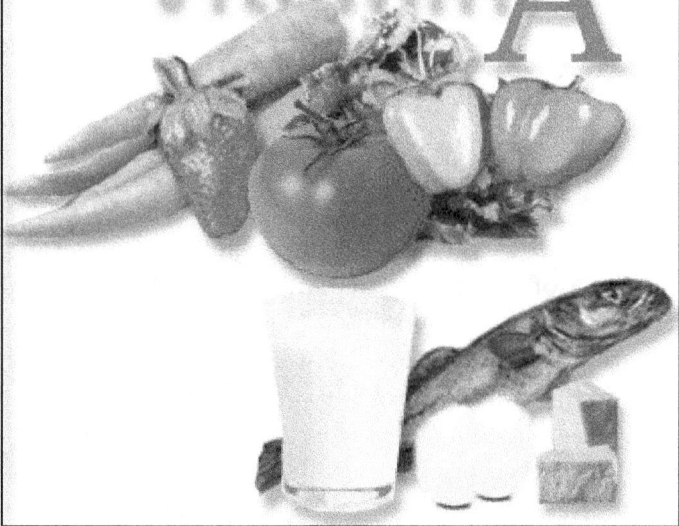

CHAPTER 19

Eating Vitamin A Foods

Vitamin A is a fat-soluble vitamin, although technically it can be either water-soluble or fat-soluble depending on the source. The active form of vitamin A is called Retinol and is the fat-soluble form. There is a pre-cursor to vitamin A, a carotenoid like beta-carotene that is water-soluble. Vitamin A is important for vision, especially night vision. It also repairs bones and tissue and is involved in reproduction and fetal development. It is very important to your immune system to fight off infections and diseases.

Food sources of vitamin A

Good food sources are whole eggs, milk products, and beef liver. Non-fat dairy products are fortified with vitamin A because when the fat is taken out of dairy products, you lose the vitamin A. This is because that form of vitamin A is Retinol, the fat-soluble one.

The pre-cursor, the beta-carotene with the other carotenoids are found in vegetables and fruits, in dark green, rich yellow or orange fruits and vegetables such as carrots, cantaloupes and sweet potatoes.

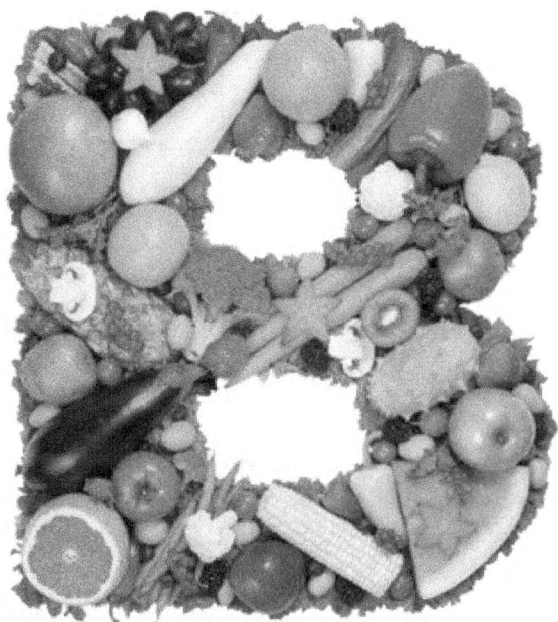

CHAPTER 20

Eating Vitamin B Foods

The B vitamins, that big class of vitamins, are all important for digestion, the process your body must go through to convert the food you eat and absorb into usable energy. All your body cells have the ability to turn your food into energy. How you move and how your body functions are all energy based. One of the many systems your cells use to release energy is called the Krebs cycle. The B vitamins are all involved in these cycles. When you are going through stressful situations that use up a lot of your energy, you need to supplement your diet with extra vitamin B.

B vitamins do some additional things. For example, thiamine (otherwise known as B1) is important for your nervous system, your heart muscles, and it regulates your appetite.

Vitamin B2 is called Riboflavin, and it plays a role in your mucous membranes and your skin.

Vitamin B 3, called Niacin, helps to improve your digestive system, your skin and your nervous system. When used as treatment, it helps to lower the bad cholesterol (LDL) by increasing the good cholesterol (HDL).

Vitamin B6 is important for your nervous system functions. It assists your body in making neurotransmitters that help nerve function. It helps your body produce the hormones Serotonin and Norepinephrine that influence mood. It also helps in the production of the hormone melatonin that regulates sleep and your body clock.

Folic acid, which is one of the most common B vitamins, helps your body turn food into energy. It reduces the risk of brain and spinal cord damage during the first few weeks of pregnancy. It ensures proper cell division and red blood cell formation. It is very important for women of childbearing age who are planning to become pregnant or who are already pregnant to consume enough folic acid to prevent neural tube deficiencies. One of the most common neural tube deficiencies is called spina bifida. Folic acid is essential to prevent it.

Vitamin B12 is different because it is not found in plant foods, only in animal foods. In addition, certain foods are fortified with it. This is important for vegans to know because they are not consuming any animal foods. They need to supplement their diet with B12, or make sure they are getting enough foods fortified with it.

Food Sources for B vitamins

In general, Vitamins B are widespread in the food supply. They are found mostly in vegetables, in many animal products such as meat, dairy, and many foods are fortified with B vitamins. There is another B vitamin that is a little more difficult to get, and that is vitamin B12.

CHAPTER 21

Eating vitamin C foods

Vitamin C, a water-soluble vitamin, is also known as ascorbic acid. It protects against the harmful effects of free radicals that can damage our cells, so vitamin C is known as an anti-oxidant. For instance, if you cut an apple in half and leave it out in the open, it turns brown rather quickly. That is because the exposure to oxygen in the air damages its cells. Since our bodies are exposed to oxygen, it can cause damage to our cells as well. Not only does oxygen cause a problem, the toxins that we are exposed to damage our cells, causing oxidation. Some of these toxins are cigarette smoke, toxins in the air and chemicals. Vitamin C also acts as an anti-oxidant. If you put lemon juice on top of the apple, you will notice that it will take much longer to turn brown, or might not turn brown at all. This is because vitamin C is one of the components of the lemon juice protecting the flesh of the apple. Vitamin C also assists in the formation of collagen, important for healthy gums and the development of bones and teeth. It is needed for wound healing. Vitamin C helps resist infections; it is also used to treat the common cold. It has been found to help decrease the risk of cancer and possibly heart disease. Vitamin C acts as anti-histamine; it reduces excess mucous production, helps to reduce sneezing and itchiness of the eyes. It can also be used to prevent those symptoms.

Food sources for Vitamin C

Common food sources include fruits and vegetables; particularly, bell peppers, kiwis, oranges, broccoli, strawberries, tomatoes, watermelon, potatoes, bananas, carrots. Therefore, vitamin C is obviously pretty widespread in our plant supply.

Vitamin D

The body makes vitamin D when it
is exposed to Ultraviolet (UV) rays from the sun.

FOOD SOURCES:

Cheese
Margarine
Butter
Fortified Milk
Healthy Cereals
Fatty Fish

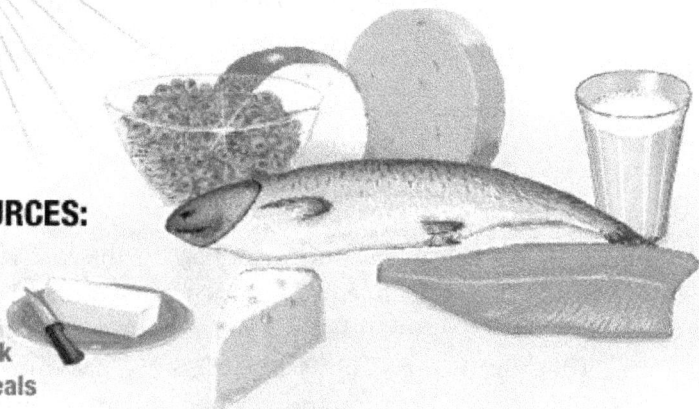

CHAPTER 22

Eating Vitamin D Food:
The Gift Of The Sun

Vitamin D is a vitamin and a hormone. In the last few years, the health industry has been learning much more about the importance of vitamin D. The recommended dietary amounts for daily intake are going up. They used to be about 400, but now the thinking is that it is too low. Most people are actually deficient in vitamin D, and the recommendations may go up to well over 1,000. This is especially true for someone who has other health risks like bone disease. Even some cancers are being connected to low levels of vitamin D.

Vitamin D is our sunshine vitamin because we get it from the sun. It is different from other vitamins as it is also a hormone in the body. Our skin cells absorb the sunlight and convert it to a usable form of vitamin D in the body. Many people are becoming deficient due to the overuse of sunscreen and the fact that many of us work inside, never setting foot outside for some sunshine. Obviously, it is important to use sunscreen to prevent skin cancer. However, sunscreen is now in everything we put into our body. While that is good for reducing our skin cancer risk, unfortunately it is causing deficiencies in vitamin D because we are not absorbing it from the sun. The new research is showing that vitamin D is needed to prevent many forms of cancers. We avoid the sun to prevent one form of cancer, whilst becoming deficient in vitamin D that helps prevent other cancers. It is a catch-22 situation.

Vitamin D helps maintain the calcium and phosphorous levels in your body; it increases their absorption into your blood stream. Calcium and phosphorous are needed to develop and maintain your bones and teeth, so vitamin D is essential. It also prevents deformative diseases such as rickets in children and osteomalacia in adults. Vitamin D deficiency leads to poor bone formation in children and then bone loss in adults.

Vitamin D assists immune functions and cellular growth. It is involved in fetal development. As mentioned, deficiency in Vitamin D has lately been connected to many different cancers.

Food sources of Vitamin D

Although the primary source is the sun, you also get vitamin D through fatty fish such as cod-liver oil, salmon, tuna, sardines and mackerel. Milk and dairy products are typically fortified with vitamin D, and you can find it in egg yolk and beef liver. This means the sources are limited for vegetarians and vegans.

Since it is essential to get vitamin D through exposure to the sun, we need to get a good 15 minutes of sun exposure a few times a week on our arms and our face. If you cannot do that, and if you are not getting enough in your diet it is important to supplement with vitamin D. It is particularly important in darker skin people living in countries that have poor sunshine.

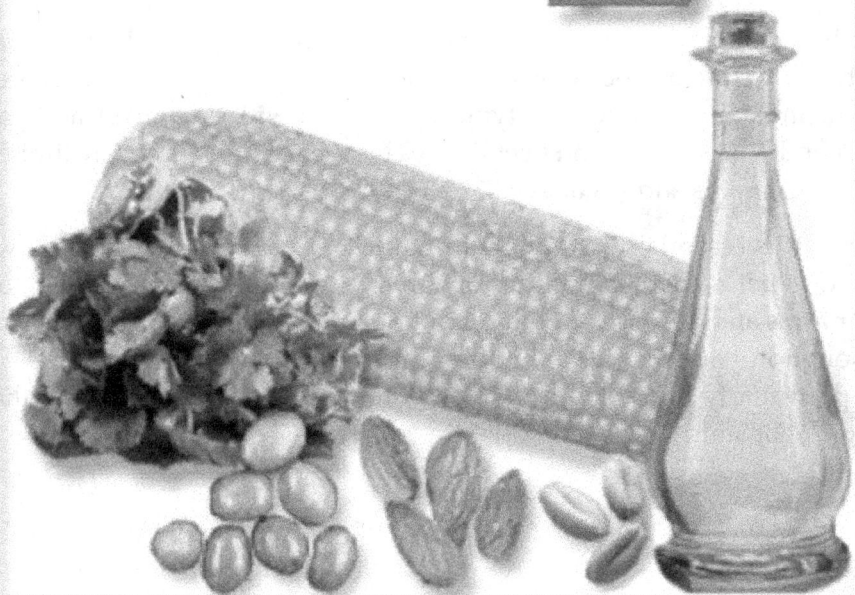

CHAPTER 23

Eating Vitamin E Foods

The next fat-soluble vitamin is vitamin E. Vitamin E is another of those acting as an anti-oxidant, a scavenger of free radicals that helps prevent damage to our cells. Vitamin E has also been connected to preventing cardio-vascular disease and some cancers. It contributes to our immune system function and is involved in DNA repair.

Food sources for Vitamin E

Best sources for vitamin E are wheat germ oil, fortified cereals, green leafy vegetables, some nuts, legumes and whole grains.

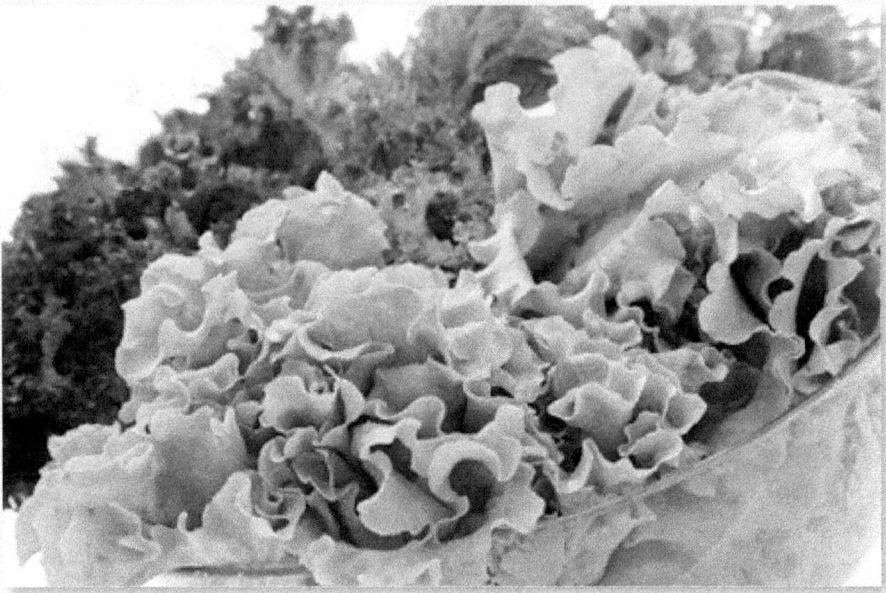

CHAPTER 24

Eating Vitamin K Foods

Vitamin K, also a fat-soluble vitamin, is essential for blood clotting profile. Forming blood clots is important to prevent over bleeding from wounds and internal bleeds. Vitamin K is involved in the synthesis of bone proteins as well.

Nevertheless, our body can also synthesize some vitamin K. The bacteria in our large intestine can synthesize vitamin K, and we absorb it from our large intestine. It does not produce enough to give the body all it needs, so it is partially essential because we can only make some of it.

Food sources for vitamin K

Vitamin K is widespread in the diet; it is found in green leafy vegetables. It is also found in beef liver, but to a lesser extent. It is found in milk, meat, eggs, cereals and other fruit.

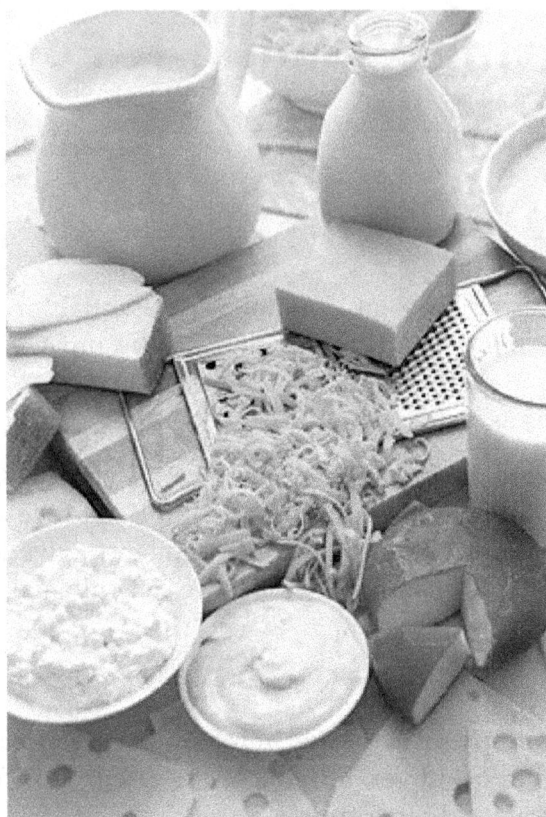

CHAPTER 25

Eating Calcium-Rich Food

Calcium is involved in our bone and teeth structure, but it does more than that. It aids muscle contraction, is important for blood clotting and for blood vessel constriction and dilation. It is involved in the secretion of enzymes and hormones, and plays a role in our nerve system function.

Calcium prevents bone leakage and bone weakness. It works on your cellular channels preventing hypertension. In addition to that, there is some connection to calcium in high cholesterol, calcium in diabetes, colon cancer and obesity. Therefore, it is important to get enough calcium in your diet.

Food sources for Calcium

Calcium is widespread in foods. Most people assume that dairy is the number one source. Dairy does contain calcium, but we do not always absorb it from dairy. It is not necessarily the best source to use for your calcium intake. It is also found in dark green leafy vegetables such as kale, Chinese cabbage, broccoli, mustard and turnip greens, Bok Choy, parsley, watercress and even some seaweed. You can also find calcium in canned fish with little bones, canned salmon or sardines that have edible bones. Certain foods like juices, soymilk and cereals are fortified with Calcium. Tofu is typically processed with calcium, so you can get it that way as well. Almonds and almond milk products are another source of calcium.

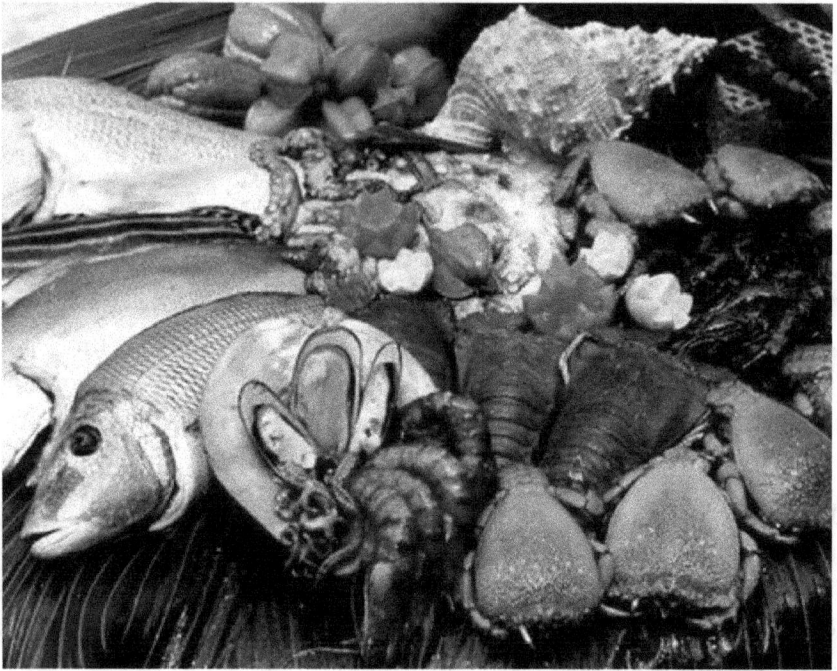

CHAPTER 26

Eating Iodine-Rich Foods

Iodine is a very important mineral used by the thyroid in the production of thyroid hormone. The thyroid hormone regulates your metabolism. It is your best friend when it comes to weight loss. A poorly functioning thyroid leads to low thyroid hormone production that then slows down your metabolism. With a slow metabolism, you gain weight easily and have a hard time losing it. Unfortunately, many people have malfunctioning thyroids but are not aware of the problem. We just adapt and live with it. Signs of low thyroid functions are fatigue, constipation, weight gain, dry skin, dry hair, hair loss hair and brittle nails.

One of the quickest ways to help your thyroid and eventually your metabolism is to ensure you consume adequate iodine. The iodine content of table salt is just enough to prevent deficiencies. Thyroid deficiency often leads to swelling in your neck called goiter. You need adequate Iodine to prevent that from happening. Children can get mental and physical retardation with Iodine deficiency, and a condition called cretinism.

Food sources for Iodine

Foods that contain or include iodine are iodized sea salts. You can also find it naturally in seafood, iodine fortified breads and dairy products.

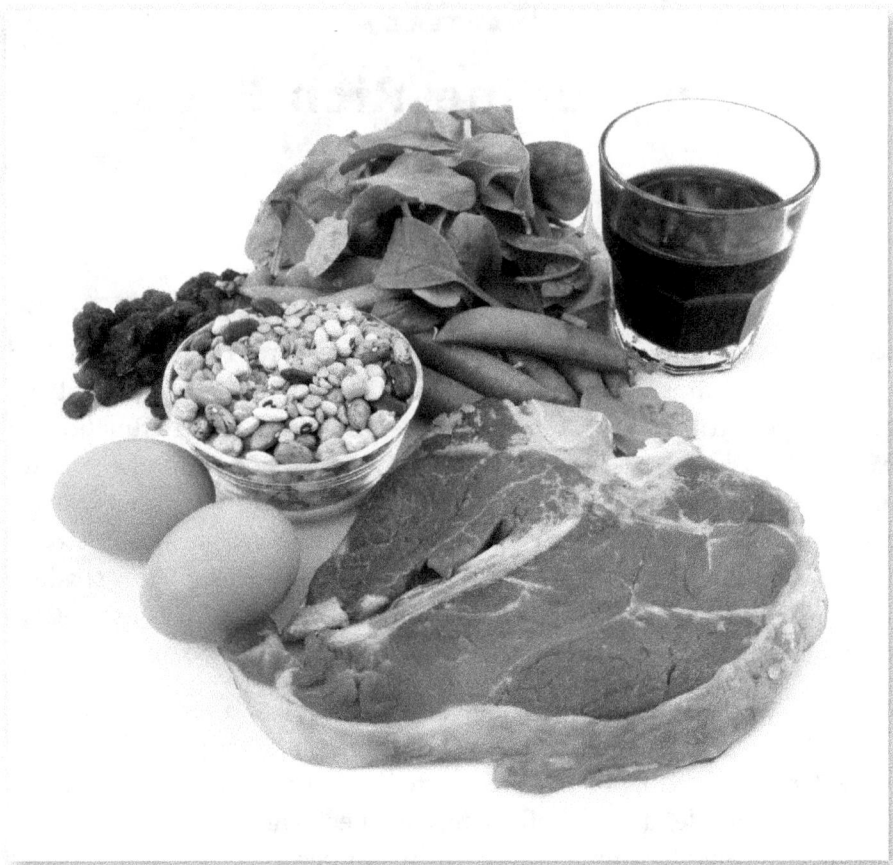

CHAPTER 27

Eating Iron-Rich Foods

Your red blood cells are involved with transporting oxygen throughout your body. They need iron to function properly. When oxygen is adequately transported to your cells, they can get on with energy production, and you feel good. If oxygen transportation is deficient, then you feel sluggish and tired with very low energy levels. Although iron is a trace mineral, it is an important one. It is needed for the formation of hemoglobin in your red blood cells and myoglobin in your muscle. These are involved in how our body carries oxygen to your cells. Iron is involved with energy metabolism, and the immune system. It helps regulate cell growth, and we need it to prevent iron-deficiency anemia.

Food sources for Iron

There are two sources: animal and plant. We absorb better the iron from animal foods. Animal sources include red meat, organ meat, some fish, some poultry and eggs.

There are ways to increase the absorption of plant iron. One of them is with vitamin C. When you consume a vitamin C source with an iron plant source, you improve the absorption. The other way is to cook in cast-iron pots. You can cook something that simmers for a long time, like soups, stews or tomato sauces (the more acidic the better). The food you cook will absorb the iron from that cast-iron pot, and we then consume it. This does not do a great deal for someone who is anemic and wants to focus on plant foods, but is helpful. Plant sources include beans, lentils, whole and enriched grains, green leafy vegetables and some dried fruits.

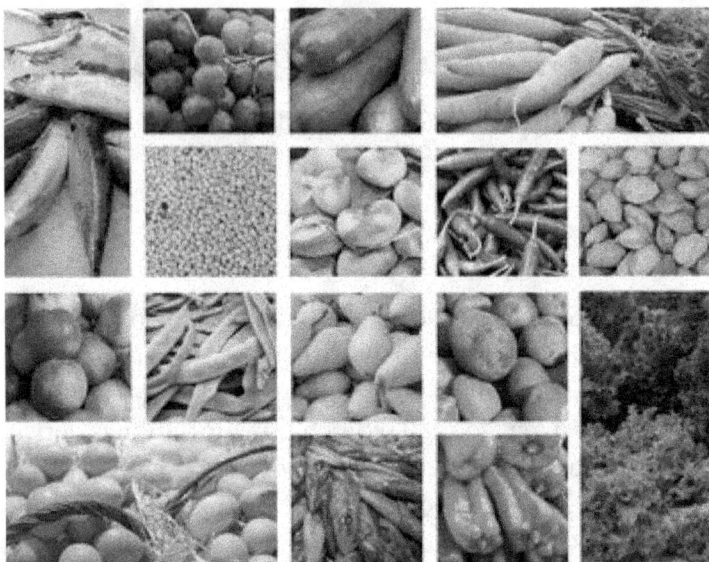

CHAPTER 28

Eating Magnesium-Rich Foods

Magnesium deficiency is the most common deficiency today. It is assumed that we all have had a deficiency of magnesium at some point. First, magnesium is important for the well functioning of your nerves and muscles. It is involved in energy metabolism and helps control your blood sugar levels. It is involved in muscle contractions and blood clotting. Magnesium is part of your bones and your teeth. It supports your immune system. It helps prevents hypertension, diabetes and some heart disease. The other quite important thing about magnesium is that it helps prevent constipation. Many people suffer from constipation, especially those with low fiber diets. It helps to improve the muscle contraction of your colon and gets your feces moving better. If you have constipation and have tried to increase the fiber and fluids in your diet without success, try magnesium.

Food sources for Magnesium

Food sources include green leafy vegetables, legumes, nuts, seeds, whole grains. Some water or hard tap water has magnesium in it.

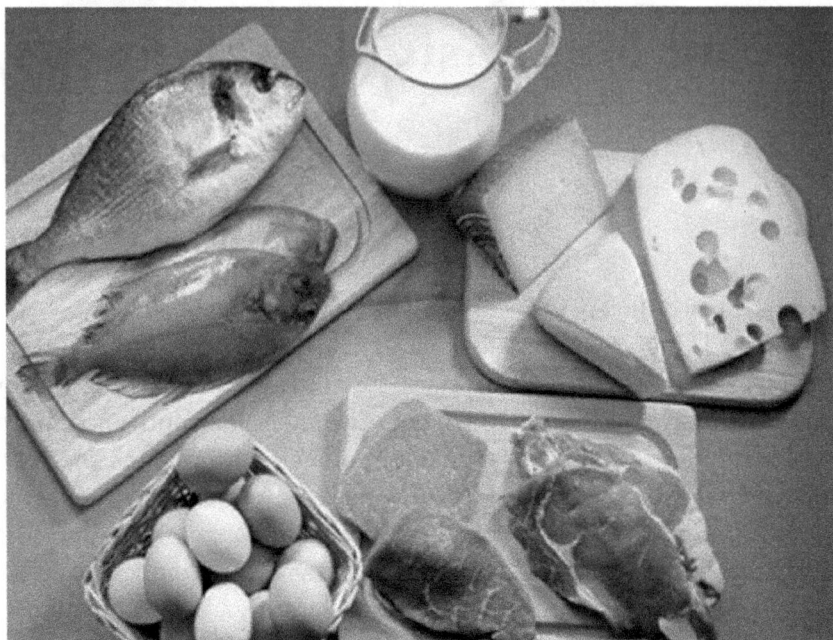

CHAPTER 29

EATING PHOSPHOROUS-RICH FOODS

Phosphorous is important for both bone and tooth structure. It is part of our DNA and RNA that has to do with cellular growth. It is essential for energy metabolism, and it activates some B vitamins. There is phosphorous in all animal and plant cells; therefore, phosphorous deficiency is quite rare.

Food sources for Phosphorous

It is very high in meats, poultry, eggs, fish, milk, legumes and whole grains.

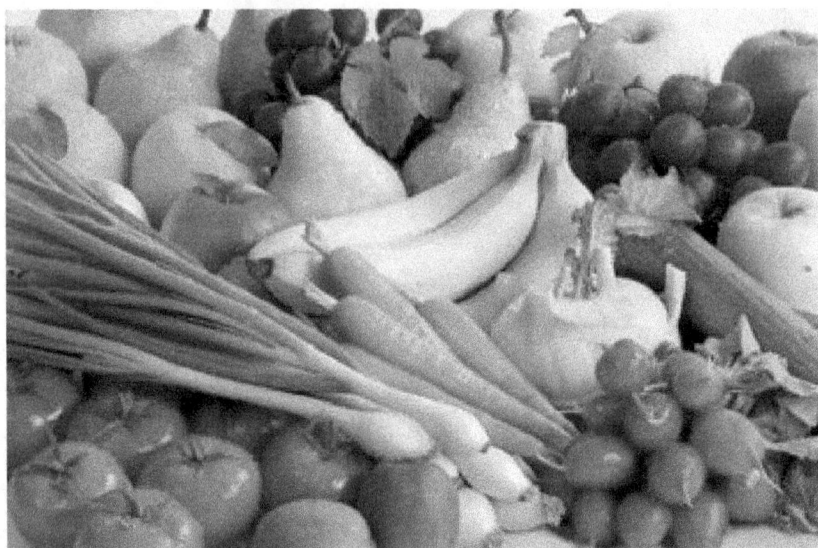

CHAPTER 30

Eating Potassium Rich Foods

Potassium is one of our electrolytes. It helps maintain our water and electrolyte balance. You need to have enough potassium to ensure cellular hydration and stability. The other electrolytes are sodium, magnesium, chloride and calcium. They are electrolyte substances that conduct electricity in the body.

Potassium is an important mineral for the proper functioning of all cells, tissues and organs. Its most critical function is the well-being of our heart, muscle health and nervous system. For someone with kidney disease, it is difficult to regulate potassium. This is dangerous because too high or low potassium can lead to heart failure.

Food sources for Potassium

Potassium is found in all animal and food products, so deficiency is rare. It is very high in fresh unprocessed foods, vegetables, fruits, some meats, dairy, legumes and grains.

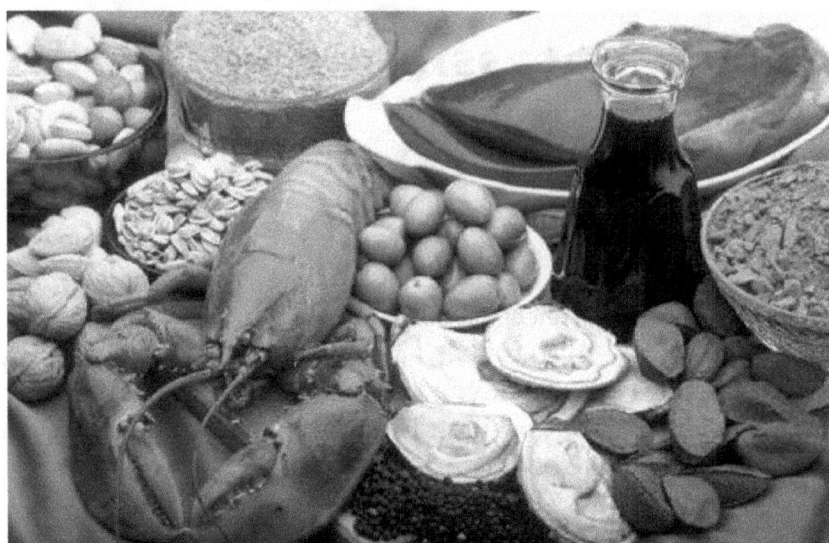

CHAPTER 31

Eating Selenium-Rich Foods

Selenium is an interesting mineral because it is the only one that also acts as an anti-oxidant, like vitamin C. Selenium also helps regulate thyroid function and assists in our immune system function. Some research connects selenium with decreased risk to certain cancers.

Food source for Selenium

It is better to supplement Selenium because its presence in foods depends 100% on soil content. Some parts of the world are depleted of selenium (New Zealand is one). There is selenium in meat products, chicken, seafood, fish, and eggs. Brazil nuts are rather high, also some grains, garlic and mushrooms.

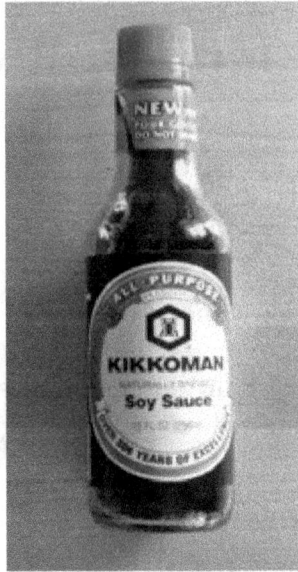

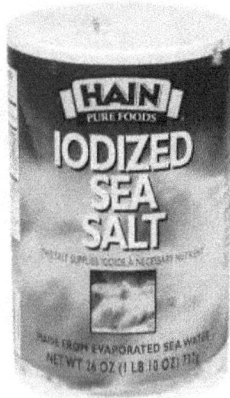

CHAPTER 32

Eating Healthy Sodium

Sodium is another electrolyte mineral, essential for regulating our water balance. It has also required for nerve and muscle activity, and necessary for acid base balance, helping with the absorption of water and some other nutrients in the body.

Food sources of Sodium

The best source of healthy Sodium is Sea salt. However, in today's world, the primary source of sodium in our diets is processed foods. Anything that is packaged, boxed or canned, typically has sodium in it. Table salt is another source. Sodium is present in soy sauce, also in natural foods such as seaweed.

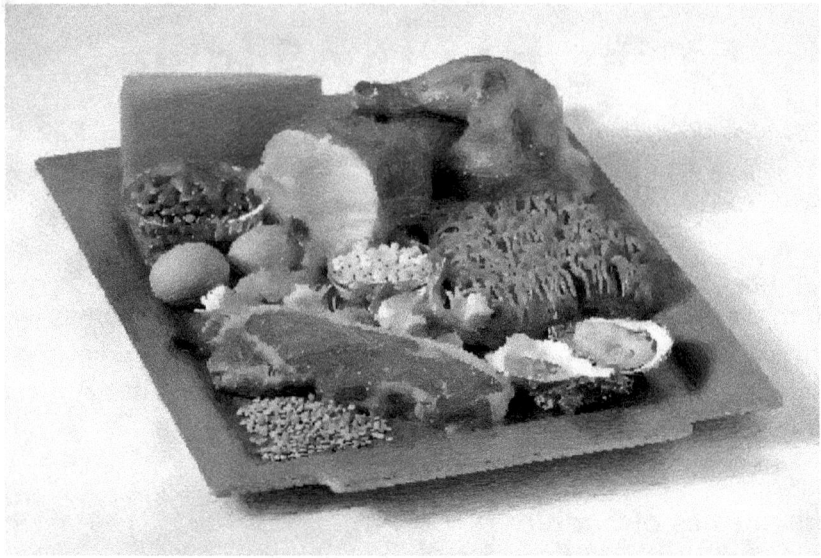

CHAPTER 33

Eating Zinc-Rich Foods

Zinc assists in the action of enzymes in your body. It is essential for immune system function and important for wound healing. There is a connection to zinc in insulin production and in thyroid function. Zinc is found in meat, poultry, seafood, eggs, dairy, whole grains, fortified cereals and legumes.

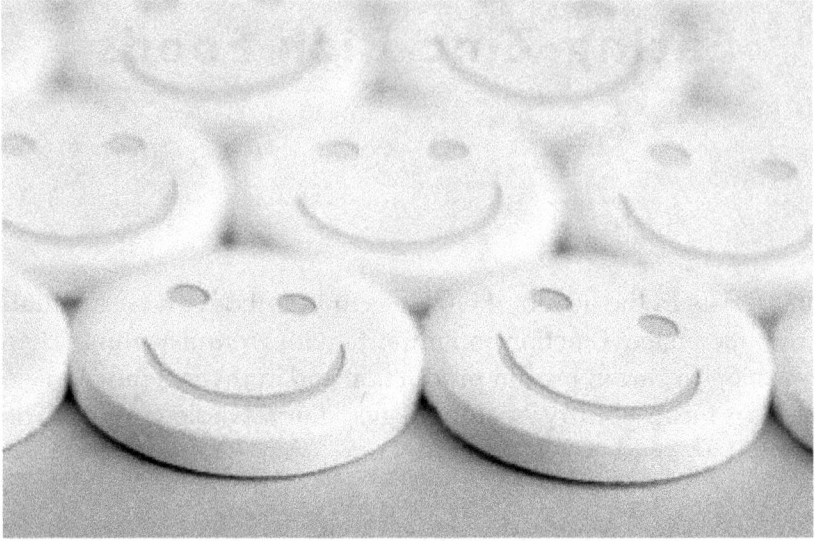

CHAPTER 34

To Supplement Or Not To Supplement

As a doctor, I am often asked by clients if they should supplement vitamins and minerals. My answer is "maybe." It depends on you. If you can be sure that your diet is varied enough to include all that the body needs, then you do not need to supplement.

However, if you are like the rest of us who do not get enough of the nutrients from our daily diet, then yes, you should supplement. My point is that supplementation is a personal choice, not one that a doctor will make for you. You have to take this responsibility. The point of supplementation is to give you more health, more energy, and more wellness. Therefore, it is truly up to you.

Realistically, it depends on what we eat, how much of what we eat, where do we get our food from, how far that food has traveled, how processed is that food, how have we cooked that food, how long has it been sitting on the shelf or in our refrigerator. All of these things matter in the nutrient content that your body absorbs from that food.

Most people probably do not get all their needs met every day. Our needs change daily, so it is important to consider that. For that reason, I typically recommend a general multivitamin for most people. If someone does not want to take vitamins, I do not think it is essential to do so, for someone who really wants to, a good general multivitamin is probably helpful.

You definitely should buy supplements that are suitable for your age and gender, because they are not all appropriate for everybody. For example, men should not be supplementing with iron unless instructed by a doctor. Women of childbearing years, and women who want to become or are already pregnant need additional folic acid, vitamin D, calcium and iron. They should be on pre-natal vitamins to get those nutrients. Someone who is a vegan should supplement with B12. They also may want to consider calcium, vitamin D and zinc, depending on what their diet is like. There are many different reasons to take supplements or not to take supplements.

Then there is the question of taking separate supplements or taking a multi-supplement. I think that in general the best way to start is a multi-vitamin because it has a good amount of everything, and you can add on from there. Certain vitamins are not going to be high enough in the multi-vitamin. Calcium is a good example of that. Your body does not absorb calcium in large doses. They never put enough calcium in a multi-vitamin, not more than 40-50 grams, definitely not enough. Therefore, if your diet is not high enough in calcium, you will want to supplement separately with calcium once you are used to taking a multivitamin.

You will probably also want to supplement separately with vitamin D if you do not have 15 minutes a day to spend in the sun. You may live in an area that has a long winter or where it is very cloudy or rainy. Maybe you do not get outside for a lot of sun. Then vitamin D is probably something you are going to be deficient in.

In addition, it depends in your health status. If you have iron-deficiency anemia, you will want to supplement with iron. Iron supplementation can sometimes need to be taken with food. It depends on which ones you chose. However, multi-vitamins generally can be taken with or without food. It is better to take them with food and can be taken morning or night. Your body will often excrete what it doesn't need, especially the water-soluble vitamins.

If you are taking B-complex vitamins, your urine may look bright yellow or even orange. That is a reaction from how your body processes the vitamin.

There are many companies that sell vitamins. An all-natural, food-based one is best. There are synthetic vitamins as well that will do just fine. I advise clients to get their supplements from health food or organic food stores. If you are buying a multivitamin from the local shops, then you need to avoid the tablets that look "well-done" like a painted wall.

You want to buy tablets that look like dirt, as if they are not completely done. A tablet that looks like dirt or the ground look is better for you.

It is not the content that is so terrible; it is rather a question of how it is bound together. There are many binders in vitamins, and your body needs to break down them down in order to absorb them. I have found that the cheaper the vitamin, the less we actually absorb of its content.

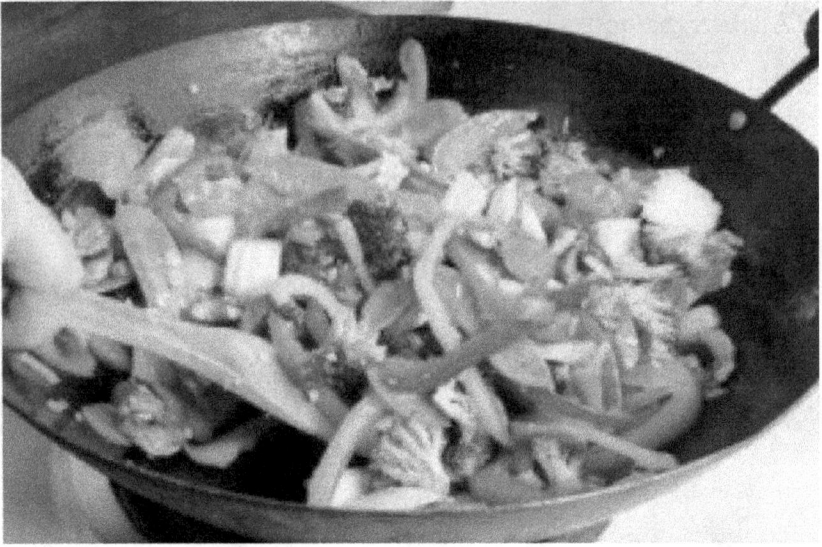

CHAPTER 35

Simple And Healthy Cooking

The good thing about simple cooking is that it can be as much fun as you want it to be. You can do an activity by yourself or with other people. It can be relaxing and therapeutic if you let it. You can listen to your favorite music or watch your preferred TV show while cooking.

You can have an aromatherapy oil burner switched on to provide a relaxing atmosphere as you are chopping and dicing the vegetables. You can cook while chatting to friends or a lover. For me, cooking is therapeutic. I do it in a way that brings out even more joy in my life.

I cook with music on, and I dance while doing it. I also watch music videos. This way cooking does not become a chore. I advise you to find ways to incorporate fun activities into your cooking routine. It has to be done, so it might as well be enjoyable.

As a parent, you can involve your kids with less dangerous tasks in the kitchen as you cook together. Kids love to do this, so start them from a young age. Make them wash the veggies, toss the salad, or set the table. They can pick their favorite condiment and put it on the table.

Cooking can be your private time too. It can be "Me time." It can be a spiritual time for you to connect to yourself. While cooking you can appreciate the food as you prepare it. Appreciate the fact that you have food to cook, its color, its texture, the ground it grew in, and the farmer who farmed it.

You can go as deep as you want with your gratitude as you are cooking. This can be your time to gift yourself, YOU.

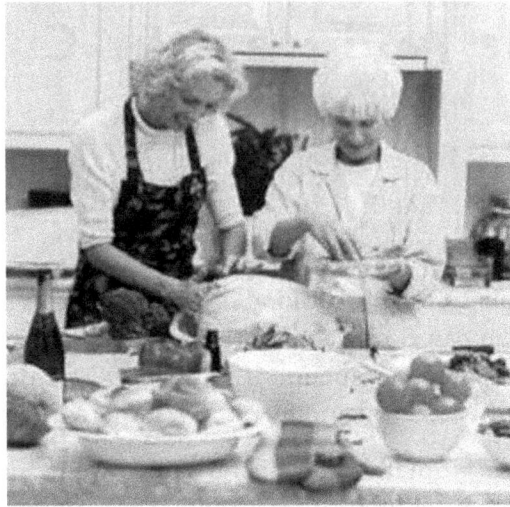

CHAPTER 36

How To Prepare Food In Advance

If you are living alone, I advise you to invest in a large fridge with a larger freezer. This allows you to prepare meals in advance and freeze them. It is a great way to get rid of the "I don't have time" excuse. Cooking is one of the easiest things to do if you are prepared in advance.

A large fridge allows you to buy many healthy foods at once and keep them handy. Fill up your fridge with fruits and quick to eat vegetables such as cucumbers and carrots to snack on. Use those pretty zip bags and lay them flat in your freezer to save space.

Another idea if you live alone or get bored with cooking is to cook with friends. You can find what I call a cooking buddy with whom you exchange food once you have cooked it. This will give you a bit of variety instead of eating the same food all the time.

You cook a large meal one day and share it with them. Then they cook a large meal two days later and exchange with you. This gives you enough food for a week with minimal effort, plus the bonus of variety. If you had four friends as your cooking buddies, you arrange between the five of you to each cook a meal for five people.

Then you exchange the meals between the five of you. All of you have to do is cook just one meal large enough for five people, but in return get five different healthy home-cooked meals for the week with no effort at all. This is a great alternative to junk foods.

You can chop veggies while watching a relaxing movie on a Sunday, and then cook it and freeze it. If you have a loving family or a partner to cook with, the experience becomes even better. Most people do not like the idea of spending time cooking, but this method spares you time and allows you to bond with your friends.

TiPS

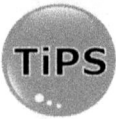

Cooking quick healthy meals:

There are many ways to make quick and healthy meals that do not take up your time. When you come home hungry after a long day at work, the last thing you want to do is hang around in the kitchen cooking. Here are some ideas of fast healthy meals.

Make a 1-pot meal

Make brown rice in the rice cooker. This is effortless because all you have to do is put in the brown rice and salt, switch on the cooker and get on with your life.

You can also use a slow cooker. All you have to do is drop in your meat and flavorings in the morning before going to work, turn it on and the food will be ready when you get home. Then you just add a tossed salad. This is such a quick method that I am surprised that few people do it. Dinner is ready for you as soon as you get home. It is a wonderful feeling to walk into your house and smell the aroma of a home-cooked meal. With this method, you have a healthy meal that is quicker to make than fast food takeaways. The waiting time at the fast-food place becomes longer than the salad tossing time.

Stir-fry

The trick to a good stir-fry is to chop the vegetables in advance. Place them in clear containers and store in your fridge. Chopping the vegetables can be done on your day off. You can also use frozen chopped vegetable. Stir-Fry is just a matter of adding the ingredients together and quickly cooking them, but you need a good wok. Remember to take the meat out of the fridge in the morning, so that it is defrosted by the time you get home. It does not matter what combination of vegetables and meat you use; stir-fry will always taste good.

Vegetable roast

Another way to use vegetables is to chop them into bigger chunks and then freeze them. Later, you can re-heat them up when you want to eat or are in a hurry. You can use the oven or a small toaster oven for a fast dinner. Put them into the oven as soon as you walk in the door. Then, while the dinner is cooking, you can change and relax.

Frozen vegetables

Frozen vegetables have a lot of the original goodness in them and are a great backup plan for quick meals. They are great alternatives to fresh vegetable. They are already chopped and are easy to use in a healthy meal straight away.

Whole-grain and beans

These are good foods to keep around, and are interchangeable. You can cook a large pot of them at the beginning of the week. Then you can eat them with different things to change the flavor. You can have them for dinner, use them as porridge for breakfast, add them to a pot of soup, to your stew, or even add a scoop to the salad you take for lunch.

Healthy soups

These come in handy in the winter and are easy to make.

Omelets

They are quick to make after work. Add chopped veggies to the eggs and eat with salads. This makes for an easy healthy meal.

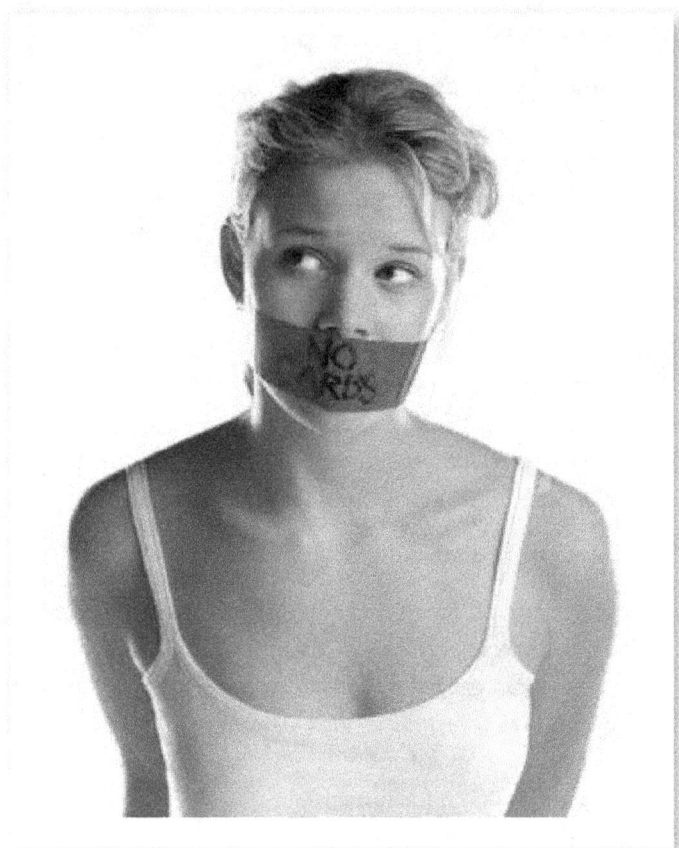

CHAPTER 37

How To Beat Your Food Cravings

There are many reasons why people will crave certain foods. Many are physiological, but there are also psychological reasons. For example, you may need a hug; you are in a job you hate, or you are not getting enough sleep. In these cases, you are definitely going to create cravings for sweet food or caffeine. You are not getting enough recuperation overnight while you are sleeping.

That means you are going to be energy deprived and will need to get it from extra foods and energy stimulants. Many times people will be drawn to non-nutritious forms of energy. One of the reasons is that foods like sugar or caffeine do not take long to be digested and absorbed. Other foods that you eat have to be chewed; they need to go down through your throat into your stomach.

They need digestive enzymes and acids to start breaking them down. Depending on how quickly that food breaks down, you will not get energy from them for perhaps 20 minutes. If you eat fruit, it could take 20 minutes. However, for most complex carbohydrates and proteins, it can take an hour before you are feeling energy from that food, 40 minutes at the least.

When you eat something that is sugary, that has a lot of sweetness to it, that food is already being digested in your mouth. You are getting energy right through your cheeks and tongue. Often a person runs low on energy, or they have not had enough calories. They might be experiencing hypoglycemia, or if they are diabetic, they might feel as though they are going to pass out.

In these cases, they are given juice or white flour, something sweet and sugary that is going to be digested and absorbed by the blood-stream quickly.

What is your guilty pleasure? Many of us have them. We just cannot do without these cravings. No matter how hard we try, we cannot seem to let go of them. Mine is ice cream. Having cravings is not a major health concern. However, it can affect your life and your health if it gets out of control. I had a client whose craving for ice cream was out of control. She would eat a 2-liter ice cream tub a day. Now, that IS a health concern.

So, what do you crave? Is it salty foods, is it something sweet or is it spicy? How about texture? Is it creamy? Is it cold, crunchy, hard, dry, or moist? All of these things will give you little hints and clues as to what is really going on in your body.

What you are craving is no accident. Your body knows what it needs, and it is always trying to find a balance. It will do whatever it takes to make sure that you are in the best shape that you can be, given the circumstances of what you are eating. Think about what time of day you are having cravings. Is it in the mornings, when you first get up? Is it around 10 or 11 o'clock, late in the afternoons, after lunchtime or in the evenings? I even had a client who used to get cravings in the middle of the night.

She would wake up and get something sweet to eat. She could not figure out why every night between 3.30 and 4.30, she would find herself in the kitchen trying to eat something. Finally, through different experiments and testing her blood sugar levels, we realized that she had low blood sugar. This meant that hypoglycemia was kicking in.

She learned not to eat sugary foods late at night and to make sure she had her dinner late enough in the evening so that she wasn't getting low blood sugar. Once she did these things, all of her symptoms were resolved.

So when you are thinking about what you want and when you want it, think about why you want it. It is not hard to figure out what and when. If someone is craving something sweet, they will know it. They will say, "I'm a sugar addict, or I love carbs, or I always want to eat sugar." It can be difficult to figure the why.

Why would someone crave something sweet? Looking at it from a dietary point of view, the reason to crave something sweet is because they already eat too much sweet or processed food. They need to add more whole foods to their diet. That will start reducing the sugar cravings.

Remember that high levels of processed carbohydrates are easily broken down into simple sugars. These are absorbed into the blood stream immediately. This spiking of glucose in the bloodstream triggers the release of the hormone insulin. The insulin pushes glucose into the cells in order to relieve the sugar high in the blood. You go from a sugar high in the blood to a sugar low. Then the body starts to crave the sweet foods.

The solution to the sugar craving is not to eat more processed carbs or sweet food; it is to eat natural carbs like sweet potatoes that have lots of fiber in them. They will not spike up your blood sugar levels.

People who crave salty things do not eat enough minerals in their diets. Salt craving is an indication that your body is craving more than just salt. People who take a lot of medications or supplements will crave salt to try to balance that in their body.

Why would people want something spicy? When people eat the standard western diet, it is not very tasty. All the flavors come from chemicals, not from the food. There is usually a lot of fat or cholesterol in the food. People tend to become overweight or stagnant.

Their blood gets thicker; circulation slows down, and they will start getting cold hands and feet. That is when they usually start craving spicy food. People often try pizza or Mexican food, things that have many added spices. The problem is that those kinds of spices can break havoc in a body that is already having symptoms of coldness.

The person is trying to create more heat inside of their body from the spices they are ingesting. Instead of eating those foods, they should eat something like a spicy marinara sauce or consistently add lower amounts of spice to their food. Cinnamon will warm them up and is a lot gentler on the system.

Are you craving creamy and cold foods? Creamy is great because most of the time when people want something creamy they want something cold. This is really an emotional food. There are physiological reasons why they might want creamy. Their bodies could be tight or dry, or they are stressed out. Creamy food can help people who are stressed, but it is usually a high mucous forming food.

I often find that people, who are wanting cold and creamy, generally in the form of ice cream, pudding or something similar, really need a hug. They are not getting enough physical attention. They do not feel appreciated for what they contribute to their family or to their job. What they need is accolades, appreciation and some physical contact.

When I get cravings for ice cream, I know it is hugging time. Therefore, if you are at my events, you will get a warm hug, baby.

Conversely, someone who craves potato chips or crackers that are salty, crunchy and dry are often angry about something. They are not in an environment where they express themselves. They cannot talk about how angry they are, so sometimes they will just munch.

Think about what it sounds like when you are chewing something that is hard, crunchy and salty. It drowns out the argument and the anger that is going on in your mind, because your mouth is making so much noise.

What if you are craving something nutritious? There will be times when you are craving something nutritious, and that is good news. Notice when this happens. It means your body is getting used to having nutrients and now, for some reason, you are not eating well. It could be just that day, or you are in a hurry, and you do not have a chance to eat the meal you would like to. I notice this when I travel because I am not always in control of my food. When I am on the road giving my seminars, I notice that the first thing I want when I get home is a home-cooked meal. I may also want something nutritious that I really love, and I am missing from my basic diet.

I remember being so happy when I started craving nutritious foods instead of junk food all the time. I hope that my readers have the chance to experience the same thing. It happens gradually and naturally. You do not have to force yourself to crave healthy foods. I do have unhealthy foods from time to time, but that is no longer the majority of times, and I thank you God for that.

TiPS

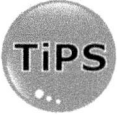

Doctor's tips for good food and digestion

1. Start by giving yourself permission to take one day off a week to relax. That day you eat whatever you want. This is the first rule I tell my clients. Start by knowing that there is an escape route and that being healthy is not a life sentence. Having an escape route allows you not to build an unconscious resistance to a healthy lifestyle. It allows you to reward yourself for being so good the whole week. It uses the principle of positive reinforcement and motivation. You can be as naughty as you want to be. You can stuff yourself and eat unconsciously as much as you want.

2. For the other 6 days, you eat consciously. This is where you relax and stay present in mind and body while you are eating. You stay conscious of what food you are putting in your body and what nutrition you are providing. You need the basic three main meals a day for your body to function well. I know you have heard this before, but I am telling you anyway. In between these main meals, you are allowed to snack, especially in the afternoons to keep up your metabolic rate that sustains you until dinner. You will not be so famished at dinner that you grab the first available thing to satisfy your hunger.

3. Proteins and vegetables (including salads) must always be part of your three main meals. Every main meal must have a protein in whatever form you like. The amount is roughly the size of your thumb or a scoop of the protein power. Your vegetables can be anything from tomatoes or mushrooms with your eggs in the morning to beans, carrots or cucumbers during the day. Just think protein with veggies at all times.

4. Nuts and seeds should be consumed with one or two of your main meals. Some people like to throw mixed seeds onto their salads or porridge. It is up to you how you want to add them to your main meals.

5. Eat your low GI carbohydrates predominantly in the earlier part of the day. Do not eat carbs for dinner, as you do not need that extra sugar boost.

6. Eat your fruits once or twice a day. You can have them as snacks in between meals, or you can add some nuts to them.

7. Drink two to three liters of water a day to maintain good digestion and wellness of the body. In some areas, you may need to boil your water to avoid the harmful effects of toxins. These toxins strip minerals from your bones and stress your liver and kidney.

8. To make this water you can drink, get two bottles of 1.5-liter size and fill them with water that you have boiled and cooled. Then keep one of those bottles by your bedside table as your bed water. You can carry the other bottle with you to drink and refill during the day. Drink the bed water the last thing before you sleep and the first thing in the morning when you wake up. If you squeeze the juice of half a lemon in the bed water, it works as a cleansing process to prepare your body for the day. Having water in your bedroom is a sure way to ensure that you will get some water into your system. I also suggest that you keep a bigger refill bottle of at least five liters in the boot of your car. You can use this to refill your 1.5-liter bottle. The message is that you need to have water readily available everywhere.

9. The next thing is to make that water taste better. You can add whatever you like so that the taste is tolerable. I suggest lemons. They are the best way to give taste to a tasteless substance. Lemon is also good as they alkalinize the body. Everything in your body needs water, even structures like bones and teeth. You are primarily water. Water is the most important substance you need to lose weight and look sexy. There are no shortcuts. Water is healing; it is soothing and frankly fabulous. So get drinking.

10. You have to avoid some foods that weaken you and do not make you feel sexy and fabulous. These are all sorts of sugars and sweetened foods. Read the labels and avoid anything that

has added sugar on its list of ingredients. Avoid any processed foods such as white rice, white salt (take natural salts such as Himalayan salts, Celtic, sea salts instead), noodles and pastas, spreads, chips and processed meats. Avoid canned foods as much as you can. Avoid deep fried foods. They are fattening; many of them contain trans-fats. They promote chronic illnesses, cancer, and they reduce the body's ability to handle blood sugar by lowering responses to insulin. Avoid non-organic dairy products from cow's milk as much as you can. Your body does not produce the enzymes necessary to digest them. It is better to use other forms of milk and milk products such as coconut milk or almond milk. Avoid alcohol; it causes decay in your body. Avoid yeast products as they increase sugar demands in your body. Avoid coffee, as it is an extra stimulant and may activate your fight and flight response, which has consequences for your internal systems.

11. Take supplements daily to make up for the extra minerals and vitamins needed for your body to function optimally. A natural way to supplement is via taking green drinks. The green drinks are usually a combination of wheat grass, barley grass, spirulina and alfalfa. These green powders are extremely well balanced in their minerals and vitamins. They alkalinize your body, and that is fantastic for people who live stressful lifestyles. You want to be careful in selecting your multivitamin supplement. You need to buy the ones that will be absorbed efficiently. Not all the cheap ones are absorbed easily. Never buy the supplement that looks bleached and over-processed. You want to buy the ones that still look muddy. They are more natural and will be more readily absorbed. Over processed ones just go through your body as expensive urine. You also need to take acidophilus and probiotics to aid food digestion. These provide a strong flora for your bowel and decrease toxic bowel metabolites. This in turn helps to keep your immune system functioning optimally. A strong bowel flora gives your liver a greater chance to detoxify the body properly.

12. Increase your intake of omega-3, 6 and 9 oils. A new scientific discovery is that children who supplement with omega-3 and

6 often experience improvement in their behavior and mood. Omega-3, 6, and 9 oils are good for you as they promote good cardiovascular health and protect against heart disease. They improve oxygen transportation throughout your body via optimizing circulation. They also help to reduce bad lipids in your body. Brain memory performance and behavioral function are improved using these oils. Omega-3 in particular may help reduce the inflammatory process in your body (gut and joints) as well as lessen premenstrual symptoms. It also has been known to increase cell membrane fluidity. Omega oils should be taken with vitamin E to reduce the risk of oxidation. These symptoms are associated with omega-3 fatty acid deficiency: poor memory, fatigue, heart symptoms, depression, mood swings, poor cardiovascular circulation, and dry skin. Many fish oils contain omega-3, 6, 9, and krill oil is potent and environmentally friendly.

13. Choose your cooking oils properly as some are loaded with Trans fats. Partially hydrogenated or hydrogenated vegetable oils should be avoided. Read the labels on your cooking oil and salad dressings. Choose the poly and mono-saturated oils, as they are healthier. These are cold press olive oil, flax seed, grape seed oil and rice bran oil.

14. Green teas are a great source of antioxidants. Drink at least 1-3 cups a day. It is refreshing and provides great fluid for the body. Berries are other great sources of antioxidants. Antioxidants are important in your weight loss journey as they help prevent the damage that occurs to cell membranes through cellular functioning. Our western lifestyles habits contribute to that process. Your cells naturally produce free radicals. These are highly reactive oxygen fragments created by normal chemical processes in the cells. Only a certain level of these free radicals is tolerable to the body. Excessive amounts are damaging. These damages to your cells can potentially cause improper functioning and increases the risk of chronic illness to develop. Antioxidants are important for liver detoxification process. Your cardiovascular system

improves with increased antioxidants in your diet. Herbs like turmeric and ginkgo are also great sources of antioxidants.

15. Digestive enzymes tablets aid your digestive system. Raw food such as fruits and vegetables provide you with natural sources of enzymes. If your level of raw to cooked food is not 50:50, then you can consider adding a daily enzyme tablet to help support your digestion. Digestion is important to ensure that the foods you are eating are being broken down to the nutrients you need. The enzymes in your body are catalysts that facilitate wellness.

16. Iodine is crucial for the internal wellbeing and functioning of your body. A deficiency in this mineral can trigger low thyroid function that slows down your metabolism. Look for a multivitamin that has added iodine in it, as many do not. White table salts that have been processed do not contain natural iodine. They have been fortified with iodine. You want to have natural salts that are not bleached white. Seaweeds are a great source for Iodine especially Kelp. Iodine forms part of the thyroid hormone that is the metabolism hormone and is necessary for good health and weight loss.

17. Have fiber in your diet. It helps digestion and wellness in the body. It gets your colon to function well.

18. Healthy foods can be made tasty with the use of condiments such as:

19. Tamari is a good alternative to soy sauce, as it has no wheat or gluten; it is lower in sodium (good for hypertensive patients)

20. Sesame oil is tasty and brings out the flavor of quinoa, brown rice and grains. You can also add it to leafy green vegetables or salads.

21. Almond and cashew butter (like peanut butter) are a great source of omega 3 fatty acids. Hemp, pumpkin and sunflower seeds are great tasting butters that give a different flavor to foods and offer alternatives to your meals.

22. Tahini can be used on bread, celery, carrots, and apples.

23. Molasses is a sweetener that is awesome for your body. It contains a significant variety of minerals that promote your health. It is a good source of Iron, manganese, copper, calcium, potassium, magnesium, vitamin B6 and selenium. You can bake with it and add flavor to cookies and cakes; it enhances beans and porridge. You can even season your chicken and turkey with it to give them a great color and a rich taste.

24. Stevia is the best sweetener alternative to sugar; it is an herb from the stevia plant. The leaves of the stevia plant taste very sweet. This sweet flavor is not due to carbohydrate-based molecules but to several non-caloric molecules called glycosides. Research has shown that a whole leave concentrate may have a direct regulating effect on pancreas and help to stabilize blood sugar levels. It is also useful in people with candida. Some treatment modalities use stevia to lower blood pressure. It is a digestive aid that reduces gas, stomach acidity and obesity. It is a good upgrade from many common sweeteners on the market that contain toxic ingredients.

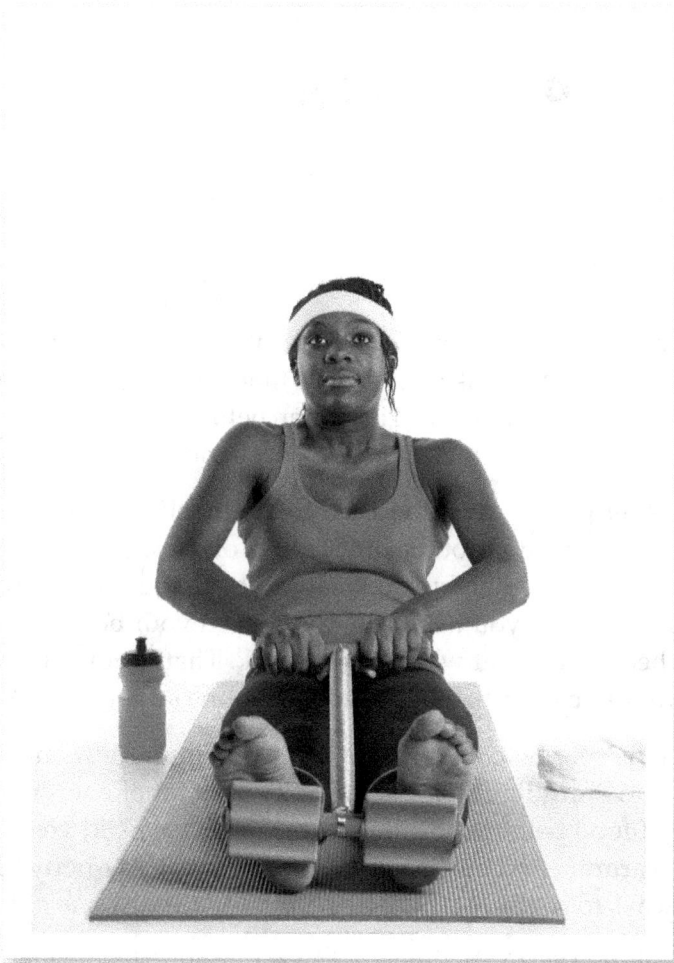

CHAPTER 38

Your Energy Levels

We have been taught that food is the only energy source for the body. Is that true? No, it is not. Why is that? Have you ever walked in nature and returned more energized than before? Have you ever been in the company of good friends and come back more energized?

Have you ever put on music and danced yourself to more energy? The answer is yes, so food is not the only source of energy for you. You need to unlearn that immediately. Un-creating the association between food and energy will help you heal from diseases in your body. Many times, you have been told to eat when you are sick. That is not true; when you are sick, your body has turned on your immune system.

It needs all its energy to be directed to your immune system rather than directing it to your digestion, which takes up a lot of energy. Stop that nonsense of food being your only source of energy. Did you know that sunlight, warmth and heat are also energizing to your body? There are so many ways to re-energize the body and food is just one of them.

Speaking of energy to the body, did you know that all these outside sources of energy are only a top-up mechanism? Your body has its own energy synthesizing mechanism that is so efficient it can light up the whole city. Each one of the 60 trillion cells of your body generates its own energy source.

This is done by the part of the cell called the mitochondria. The mitochondria in your cells produce more than enough energy for itself and for every other cell of the body. Meaning that your whole body is a raging energy machine that can support not only itself but also the while city.

The question is what are you doing to steal so much energy from your own body? Where are you getting in your own way so much as to shut down such powerful energy production? Imagine a whole city's energy being stopped by you. You are powerful, my abundant friend. So do not state, "I don't have energy," instead ask, "what can I do to bring this energy level back to its maximum?"

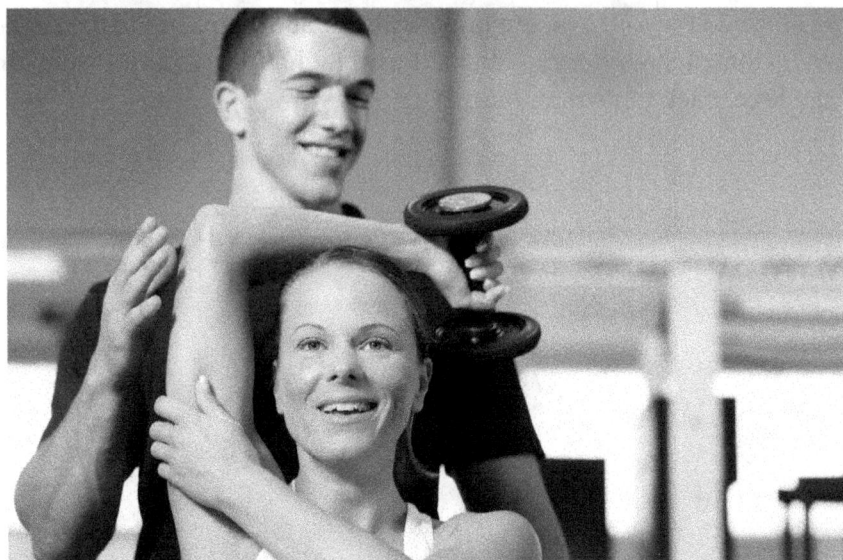

CHAPTER 39

Muscle Power And Exercise

Many people have associated exercise with failure because they have attempted exercise programs and have not been able to follow through. They have joined gyms with the bests of intentions, but have ended up wasting their money. They are paying for a contract that makes money, whether they get fit or not.

I think gyms should leave you alone if you are not using their facility. In addition, people collect workout videos that decorate their shelves or exercise books and magazines that collect dust. So what is it about exercising that produces such bad results? Why do so many of us start and yet just a few of us do it regularly?

I think exercise regimes fail because they are marketed on a false assumption that one exercise fits all. Not one type of exercise fits everyone. When you go to the gym, they give you a fake "personalized" program. It is based on what they offer in the gym, and it looks just like the program they gave to someone else who just joined. And what about those advertisements for exercise machines you see on RV?

They show a sexy woman and a man. They tell you how it only takes 20 minutes a day, 3 days a week for them to look like that, and you can do it too. They tell you this machine will fit you and your style just fine. The problem is that those machines and gym programs are good, but their umbrella approach that one exercise fits all is wrong.

Therefore, you are set up for failure before you even start. The truth is that exercising is simply you moving your body to promote better circulation. Exercise is just movement.

Like many of you, I have been there, tried that. I have decided I hate that word exercise. I chose to refer to it as me moving my butt. Your exercising style is just as unique and individual as you are. There is no such thing as an exercise approach that suits all.

Just because your cousin had great results with Pilates does not mean that you will. Being able to do an exercise routine depends on many other factors. It is not just copying what your friends are doing, or buying the latest machine.

Think about those sexy people in the advertisements, they are people who have been working in the fitness industry for years. They are not slobs who need to lose weight, so do not believe them.

Pick an activity that moves your body in a way that is enjoyable for you. That is the only way that you are going to keep it up. If you like dancing, then dance, or join a dance group. If you like to walk, then walk and enjoy the beautiful scenery. If you like boxing, then take up boxing.

Any movement you do is good for you and good for your circulation. The bonus of enjoyment will ensure that you do it regularly. You also need some resistance training, so find easy and fun ways to incorporate some weight training into your day.

I find the Swiss ball and kettle bells get you there quicker. They are easy to use, and they have exercises that tone your many body parts all at once. You get fast results even if you only have 5 minutes a day. You can sneak the kettle bells to work and do some quick reps in between clients.

You will love your body toning so quickly. Best of all, no one will be harassing you to pay your gym membership... I love simplicity in life with fabulous sexy results.

Moving your body is not a choice, it is necessary. You never stay the same; you are growing. In your life, you are either progressing, or you are regressing in whatever you do. Your health is either improving or deteriorating. Either your fitness regime is getting better, or it is falling behind.

The relationships you have with people around you are either strengthening, or they are weakening. Either you like your job more, or you dislike it more. Your body works the same way; its internal systems do not stand still.

Air and blood are always moving in your body; your heart is always beating; brain synopsis is always taking place. There is constant communication between the brain and the systems. Nothing inside you or outside you stands still.

When you do not do something every day to improve your life and your circumstance, then you are moving in a backward direction. It is a mistake to assume that nothing is happening to your body because you are not doing anything. Your body is weakening; your muscles are losing tone; your circulation is slowing, and your digestion is not optimal.

You need to get rid of such excuses as, "I couldn't be bothered to exercise," "I don't care about exercising," "there is always time later." Instead, do the movements you like and enjoy. You need to maintain momentum and keep thinking of your internal systems benefiting from the movements. Moving your body is not just for losing weight. It is for staying alive and living life to the fullest.

Movement is essential for maintaining peak health, fitness and wellness. Moving your body is anti-aging as it helps you maintain strength and tone for longer. If yoga is your thing, then do yoga.

If swimming does it for you, then do that. It is your choice and is always up to you. When you do what you love, you have a higher chance of doing it regularly. It is what you do regularly that brings you greatest results.

The benefit of doing the body movement routine that you like is that it makes you happy, which is important. More benefits are that it improves fitness and stamina; it burns calories; it strengthens the cardiovascular system and lungs; it strengthens bones and muscle tones; it increases mental capacity. It is a good way to increase oxygen levels for the long term. Higher levels of oxygen to your tissues are essential in maintaining good functions.

Having low levels of oxygen delivery to tissues and cells have been shown to lead to chronic diseases. Studies show that cancer cells thrive in environments where there are low oxygen levels, and struggle to replicate when the body's oxygen levels improve.

Do not overdo exercise because it can overstrain your body and lead to too much acid production. You do not need to over exert yourself with your body movement. Start small and grow slowly. Be guided by your own intuitive wisdom. A good way to start is 20-30 minutes a day.

If you are unfit, start with fewer minutes. Start by walking a few times in your yard.   Then you can go outside. You can go to the beach and walk there in the beauty of nature and the fresh air. Whatever you do is always up to you. Just enjoy it. Your fitness regime is a priority, not just for your body but also for your mind and soul. Check out exercise DVDs, machines, books, gyms. These will provide variety and help you decide what kind of body movement you like and what is appropriate. Always take action.

It is through doing yoga that you decide whether yoga is for you or not. You cannot just decide ahead of time without doing and feeling what it does to your body. Be courageous and adventurous by approaching different exercise styles in order to pick the best. You will be doing this routine for a long time, so choose wisely.

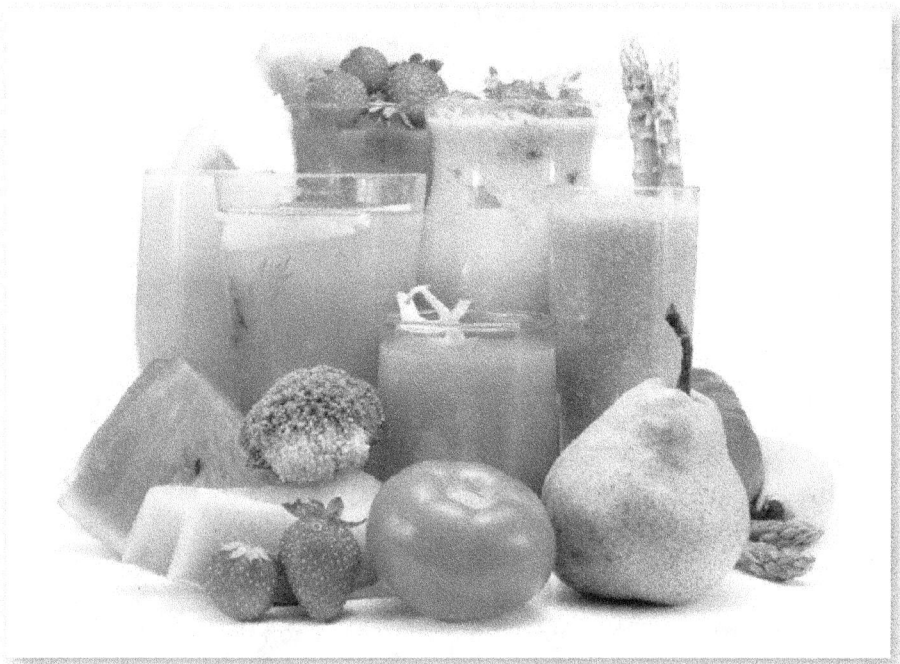

CHAPTER 40

Toxins And Detox

Detox: clean your inside as you clean your outside.

Illnesses do not come upon us unexpectedly.

They are developed from small daily sins against Nature.

When enough sins have accumulated, illnesses will suddenly appear.

—HIPPOCRATES

Detox is important. The rubbish bin in your kitchen needs to be emptied regularly in order for the kitchen to continue functioning properly. Can you imagine how badly your kitchen would look, feel and smell if you never cleaned up and emptied the rubbish bin?

There is no use in feeding the body good nutritious foods if the body's building blocks are being attacked and broken down by heavy toxic chemicals.

Every day, minimum amounts of toxins get into your body via your mouth, skin, nose, eyes and ears. They are present in the atmosphere. Detoxing is not a new invention. It is the way you function. You have organs whose entire job is to detoxify you. How can doing detoxes be a bogus thing? Your liver's job is to detox your body by getting rid of bad toxins. Your kidneys have the job of filtering your blood to clean it and rid it of its toxic contents. Your colon is a powerful waste and toxins eliminator. Under normal circumstances, your body is capable of detoxifying itself with no help from you. Unfortunately, we do not live under normal circumstances anymore. These days the detox organs are overwhelmed, and they need help from time to time. This is when doing a gentle detox program helps you.

We are overwhelmed with toxins in our lives; there is the environment that is filled with fumes from the cars and machines. Even worse, we put many toxic things into or on our bodies. Such things as chemical loaded soaps, body washes from supermarkets that have preservatives, shampoos and processed foods with more preservatives. Remember that your skin is your biggest organ, and it is absorbent. Everything you put on your skin gets into your system and is quickly absorbed. Read the ingredient list to know how many strange chemicals are used to make your supermarket body washes. What about your trusted supermarket dish washing liquids? How about your powerful stain removers, oven cleaners or your bathroom cleaners? There is a long list of harmful chemicals hidden in your supermarket products. You do not need that list of strong acids and alkaline chemicals to clean your house daily.

The following is a breakdown of many of the items you will want to stay away from. For a complete breakdown of how these chemicals are used and how they can affect our bodies, take a look at these recommendations below.

- **Diethanolamine (DEA)**:
  Shampoos, body washes, bubble bath, and shaving cream.

- **Triethanolamine (TEA)** : Moisturizers, cosmetics, deodorant, toothpaste, body oils, and washes.

- **Sodium Lauryl Sulphate (SLS)** :
  Shampoo, bubble bath, shaving foam, and cleansers.

- **Sodium Laureth Sulphate (SLES)** :
  Shampoo, bubble bath, shaving foam, and cleansers.

- **Propylene Glycol**:
  Primarily made for anti freeze for your car radiator, but surprisingly found in hand sanitizers, moisturizers, shaving creams, deodorants, and baby products.

- **Sodium Fluoride**:
  Toothpaste (though I am a mother of two and am on the fence about this one).

- **Alcohol**:
  Mouthwash, toners, and baby products.

- **Talc**:
  Baby powder, make-up, and foot preparations.

- **PABA**:
  Originally found in sunscreens but as of late has been removed from many formulations. Still make sure your sunscreen always says Paba-Free.

- **PEG**:
  Cosmetics, make-up, and shaving cream.

- **Artificial flavors**:
  Many companies use these to make things taste better and more like you would expect (the reason why Sunny D orange juice always tastes the same no matter the season), as well as toothpaste and mouthwash.

- **Artificial colors**:
  Used in many processed foods as well as make-up, toothpaste, and shampoos.

- **Benzalkonium Chloride and Benzethonium Chloride**:
  Synthetic germicides belonging to the large group of germicides known as "Quats, found in numerous household disinfectants, sanitizers including hand sanitizers and personal care products - long term use may affect immune system, cause asthma and should be especially avoided if you have COPD, or any other form of pulmonary disease.

- **Ether**:
  Nail treatments, shampoo, and conditioner.

- **Coal Tars**:
  Shampoo, conditioner, hair dyes, soap, skin care and cosmetics.

- **Aluminum**:
  Thankfully this is mostly just used in antiperspirants as larger concentrations of it have correlated to Alzheimer's.

- **Acetone**:
  Nail polish remover.

- **Formaldehyde**:
  Antiperspirants, nail treatments, and perfumes. The most interesting thing about this chemical is that was used to embalm corpses in the past but even that industry has seen how toxic the use of it was and no longer uses it.

- **Fluorocarbons**:
  Hair spray used to have a great deal more of them in it (the reason why it used to make you cough). Recently there has been a crack down on this.

- **Dioxins**:
  Shampoo.

- **Petrolatum or Mineral Oil**:
  Baby products, washes, and moisturizers.

- **Sodium Hydroxide**:
  Soaps and detergents, is a caustic poison and very corrosive to skin.

- **Triclosan**:
  Anti-bacterial soaps, hand sanitizers and even toothpaste. Its use is so widespread that it is being linked to lowering the immune system and is now being detected in breast milk. (Overuse of hand sanitizers with Triclosan is not good for your children)

This harmful ingredients list is not exhaustive and these ingredients may be found in numerous other personal care products than those listed on this page. Be sure to check your labels carefully!

- Acrylate
- acid orange 3
- Acrylate copolymers
- amorphous silicates
- Benzyl acetate
- blue 1,2,4

- bromonitrodioxane
- bronopol
- bronopol (2-bromo-2-nitropropane-1, 3-diol)
- butyl benzylphthalate
- Butylated hydroxyanisole
- butylated hydroxytoluene
- Ceteareth-3
- chlorhexidine
- Choleth-24
- chrystalline silica
- coal tar dyes
- DEA
- DEA-Cocamide & Lauramide & Oleamide condensates
- DEA-cocamide/lauramide condensates
- DEA-MEA/Acetame
- DEA-Sodium lauryl sulfate
- diaminoanisole
- diaminophenol
- diaminotoluene
- diazolidinyl urea
- Diethanolamide-cocamide, lauramide & oleamide condensates
- dioctyl adipate
- disperse blue 1
- disperse yellow 3
- DMDM-Hydantoin
- ethoxylated alcohols
- ethyl alcohol
- fluoride
- formaldehyde
- glutaral

- green 1,2,3
- hydroquinone
- Imidazolidinyl urea
- lanolin
- Laureth's
- Methacrylate copolymers
- Metheneamine
- methylene chloride
- Morpholine
- nitrophenylenediamine
- Nonoxynol
- Oleth's
- Padimate-O (octyldimethyl para-amino benzoic acid)
- PEG's (polyethylene glycols)
- polyoxymethyleneurea
- Polysorbate 60
- Polysorbate 80
- polyvinyl acetate
- polyvinyl pyrrolidone
- p-phenylphenylenediamine
- pyrocatechol
- Pyroglutamic Acid
- Quaternium-15
- quaternium-26
- red 4,9,17,19,22,33,40
- saccharin
- Sodium/Hydroxynethylglycinate
- talc
- TEA
- vTEA-Sodium lauryl sulfate

- titanium dioxide
- Yellow 5,6,8

Even when people become aware of the toxicity of the chemical cleaning products, they do not change to non-chemical plant based ones. They buy gloves to protect their hands. If you have figured out that the chemical cleaning products are so heavily toxic that they burn your hands, why continue with it? If it burns your hands, can you imagine what it is doing to your fragile lungs? Wearing gloves does not protect your nose from any chemicals. Wearing gloves only prolongs the problem; it covers it up.

The smell of chemical cleaning products is overwhelmingly strong. Sometimes you have to walk away from the fumes, as your body cannot take them. Once you have finished cleaning your home with these heavy chemicals you will be amazed how the smell stays around. It lingers, causing more damage as you continue to inhale the fumes.

Then there is the fact that it says, "do not ingest" on the bottle. You have used it to clean the kitchen bench, sink and taps. You may have used it to clean your bathrooms. Then, later you touch them and then touch the food you are preparing. Perhaps you wear protective gloves when you use dishwashing liquid because you feel the effect of that liquid on your hands is not good.

How can you continue using the very same thing you are protecting yourself from? You are feeding yourself and family that dishwashing liquid you fear. It would be wiser to change to a plant-based alternative that will not harm your hands in the first place.

The body washes and soaps you use are just the tip of the iceberg. When you get out of the shower and your skin is pulling and drying out so fast, that is a clue. Why should a product clean your skin by ridding it of all its moisture content?

Many soaps and body washes are loaded with chemicals that make foam. Unfortunately, that strips your skin of its natural defense against moisture loss. That is why when you step out of the shower, you are so dry and crackly, and you feel like the dry soil in the Sahara desert.

Why should having a shower, which is a natural thing, lead to an unnatural stripping of your skin moisture barriers? What about the acid in these body-cleaning agents? Do you need all those listed chemicals on your bottle just to clean your body? Many of those chemicals are only there to enhance the foaming ability of the product. They are not there for your benefit.

To my wonderful sexy ladies, here is bad news about the makeup you use. I love make up, looking good is great but looking sexy is better. Think about those new makeup lines that are the "long lasting" version. What has to happen to something to make it "longer lasting"? It has to have more chemicals.

Next time you get excited about a longer-lasting mascara or longer-lasting foundation, think twice. You also need to know that many mineral or natural make-up lines only need one natural ingredient in them to be called "natural-based" or "mineral-based". This is infuriating.

Once again, you have to practice discretion when you buy a "natural" or "mineral" make up range.

Look at the regular make-up you use daily and compare the list of ingredients against the list of things that are toxic to the body. You will be amazed to see how many "natural" and "mineral-based" make-up ranges contain toxic ingredients. Your eyes are the most sensitive, and I advise you to use the organic range make-ups with non-toxic ingredients.

When you buy make-up, take a list of toxic ingredients with you so you can check the contents. Never trust any make-up or beauty range that calls itself "natural," mineral-based or even "organic". Be your own judge. These chemicals are not good enough to be entering your body daily.

Many people point to the environmental world when the word toxin is mentioned. Now that you are reading the labels on your chemical cleaners, you realize that the enemy lives with you day in and day out. It is a good idea to start inside the home where the air is polluted daily with chemical fumes from the very things you use. Many people pay attention to global warming and the ozone layer while forgetting about the silent killers that live in their cupboards.

Make your air clean. The air you breathe most of the time is the one that surrounds you at home. If this air is loaded with chemicals, then your body is under attack daily and has to defend itself. You may think you are doing your bit to clean up the environment, but when you get home, you are greeted with your daily dose of toxic fumes and body products that are slowly destroying your body.

Everything you use from the time you wake up to the time you go to bed has some level of toxicity to your body. Now you can understand what I mean when I say toxins in our home are overwhelming to our systems. I suggest you have a look at my toxic ingredient chart and throw out all the agents in your household that contain even one of these.

Your health and well-being are worth it. It has been shown that some of those toxic chemicals are carcinogenic. Your body is poisoned with these toxic ingredients. It has to detoxify to a level and amount that it is not used to. The quantity, intensity and strong concentration of these toxic ingredients overpower your body. They slow the immune system and weaken the connections in your body.

As a doctor, I am appalled at how much misinformation and "truth-bending" is going on at your expense. Many of the self-care and home cleaning companies take your concerns and needs for natural product and use it against you. I am not happy with that "natural" label that misleads people. Just know that money talks when it comes to these big companies.

They will tell you what you want to hear in order to sell more products, even if they are not good for you. Toxic chemicals are cheap ingredients that these companies use to make their products. It makes more money sense to them. It gives them more profits. That is a good thing for them, but bad and life threatening to you.

Many of these bad toxic ingredients cause cancer and chronic diseases by disrupting the functioning of your body systems. It is up to you to take decision making into your hands. When you go shopping, always take the list of toxic ingredients with you. Have the guts to select your own ingredients, it is your precious body.

There are new and extensive studies coming out that conclude there are many toxic ingredients in everyday substances like toothpastes, face creams and shampoos. The companies that make these products will never tell you about these findings. You have to do your own detective work.

It is important to examine each and everything in your house. In order to get well and look fantastic, your body has to have an environment that promotes that. There is no point in putting effort into eating well and exercising if your body is hanging on to fat cells.

These cells protect you from the overwhelming amount of toxic attacks daily. Fat cells offer a refuge for the liver to deposit harmful toxins. Not many people realize that the body uses fat deposits as a way to lower the toxin loads in their body. If you walk around all the time with so much of that nasty stuff in your body, it will cause more damage to your cells and immune system.

Your fat cells help lower the burden a bit. This is why sometimes your body holds on to your fat. No matter what you do, it is a survival strategy, and you are in survival mode. Your body will do anything to survive, including keeping you fat when you do not want to be fat.

Never assume that you are fat because your body is punishing you. That is not always the case. The toxins in your body alter your body PH by creating an acidic medium, which is not favorable to cellular function. Your fat protects you by mopping out this effect to allow you to function at an optimal ph.

You must be aware of the daily body attack routine that is going on because of your cleaning and self-care products. You need to check the list of ingredients and throw out all the nasty toxic chemicals that cause you so much damage.

Look at everything from toothpaste and soaps to window cleaners. EVERYTHING must go. Your life is at stake. No one will care more about your well-being than YOU, so do it for yourself. I worked at a medical clinic where I saw many children with eczema and asthma symptoms.

When the family was asked to replace all the chemicals and toxins in their homes, the symptoms immediately started to vanish. Those kids looked lively and did not need the usual repeats of their medications. This was the biggest revelation for me as a practicing medical doctor.

I fell in love with wellness medicine then. It was good to watch people come out of their shells just by making some adjustments on their daily routines. So please do it for yourself. Your body will love you for it.

APPENDIX

Moringa Super-food: nature's multivitamins

A super-food as is a single plants that is full of multivitamins and minerals that are vital to the body in large quantities. These plants are grown naturally. They promote natural and healthier functioning of the human body. Moringa is one of the best Super- foods available world-wide today as it contains 90 essential vitamins and minerals in large quantities which are natural and easily absorbed by the human body. Moringa Super-food promotes and restores health and wellness faster and better than the rest of the super-foods.

In today world, life is so fast and very taxing on the body. People work hard to earn a living. Hard physical and/or mental work drains the body of nutrients and energy thereby shortening life span. Such energy consumption leads to deficiencies of minerals and nutrients in the body as the natural energy regeneration system gets exhausted in the body, hence the need for a recharge that can be obtained from natural super-foods and energy booster food products is greatly in need today. Stress as already discussed in the earlier chapters of the books is another good reason for the depletion of nutrients and energy levels in the body. This depletion leads to the need of natural nutrient supplement alimentation such as Moringa Super-food.

Natural Moringa Super-food product compares excessively above the usual nutrients standards commonly prescribed in health and wellness as follows:

- ➢ 2 times more protein than an egg
- ➢ 15 times more fiber than wheat
- ➢ 10 times more Vitamin-A than carrots

> ➢   15 times more Potassium than bananas
> ➢   17 times more Calcium than milk.

Moringa helps people to handle life & stress much better.

It supports the weight loss process by bringing the necessary vitamins and minerals into your bloodstream and hence reducing excessive appetite. It's an energy booster as it slows down the release of sugar into the bloodstream and stimulates the body to burn stored fat for fuel and hence boosting energy. The protein content of Moringa Super-food helps to tones muscles and helps in the re-shaping of muscle mass to fat ratio in the body leading to weight loss.

How to take Moringa Super-food:

Just like certain people eat cereal in the morning; some take a glass of milk; others take a walk/run to keep healthy and others do many different things on a daily basis to ensure a healthy life style. Moringa Super-food products should become part of one's life style. Moringa powder can be added to your morning smoothie together with other fruits and vegetable. It can also be taken on its own with water. For those who don't like powders, there are capsules available to satisfy your needs.

When to take Moringa Super-food:

A dosage of Moringa Super-food should be taken either in the morning or in the evening for its maximum health effects it should be taken daily. Interesting that Moringa Super-food is used in Malaysia in the production of Ice Cream to encourage health in children!

I encourage you to read up more on Moringa Super-food for yourself and purchase the products at www.Moringabetterlife.com.

More About Dr. Stephanie K

As a celebrated International Speaker...

Dr. Stephanie is an articulate International speaker on health, success, winning mind-set, self-healing, and stress management. She is an active member of the New Zealand speakers association. She has an inspiring and motivating nature that is loved and appreciated by audiences at her workshops, seminars, online webinars, and events. Her vivacious personality and vast medical knowledge make her a sought-after speaker in the fields of health and personal success. She runs public workshops, seminars and courses aimed at promoting health, well-being, and stress management. She offers various successful programs such as health and success, winning mind-set, breakthrough stress, gain success program, as well as Skyrocket Your Health for success.

As a graduate of the prestigious Pretoria University Medical School, Dr. Stephanie holds one of the most recognized medical degrees in the world. She had the privilege to work in world-renowned hospitals such as Groote Schuur hospital in Cape Town, South Africa. This famous hospital is well known as the first hospital to perform a heart transplant in the world! Always an avid student, she advanced her studies at Auckland University, where she did a Diploma in Public Health Medicine and Health Promotion. She is currently furthering her studies in natural anti-aging and regenerative medicine. This training allows her to use natural treatment alternatives in her practice.

Since 2005, she has resided in the lovely country of New Zealand working in the hospital system, and practicing as a holistic general practitioner with special interest in stress management and hormone treatments. Her passion lies in the use of natural treatments to support the body functions and organs, as this allows the body's immune system to activate its own healing process.

She believes that health is our biggest treasure on this planet and being healthy is as easy as 1, 2, 3!